THROMBIN
Its Key Role in Thrombogenesis– Implications for Its Inhibition Clinically

Edited by
Michael R. Buchanan, Ph.D.
Professor
Departments of Pathology and Surgery
McMaster University
Hamilton, Ontario, Canada

Stephanie J. Brister, M.D., F.R.C.S.
Cardiovascular Surgeon
Hamilton Civic Hospitals
Hamilton, Ontario, Canada

Frederick A. Ofosu, Ph.D.
Professor
Department of Pathology
McMaster University
Hamilton, Ontario, Canada

CRC Press
Boca Raton   Ann Arbor   London   Tokyo

Library of Congress Cataloging-in-Publication Data

Thrombin : its key role in thrombogenesis : implications for its inhibition clinically / editors, Michael R. Buchanan, Stephanie J. Brister, Frederick A. Ofosu.
p. cm.
Includes bibliographical references and index.
ISBN 0-8493-7649-1
1. Thrombin. 2. Antithrombins. 3. Thrombosis. I. Buchanan, Michael R., Ph.D. II. Brister, Stephanie, J. III. Ofosu, Frederick, A.
[DNLM: 1. Thrombosis—etiology. 2. Thrombosis—therapy. 3. Thrombosis—prevention & control. 4. Thrombin. 5. Antithrombins. QZ 170 T529 1994]
QP93.5.T4714 1994
616.1'35—dc20
DNLM/DLC
for Library of Congress 94-26483
CIP

Direct all inquiries to CRC Press, Inc., 2000 Corporate Blvd., N.W., Boca Raton, Florida 33431.

International Standard Book Number 0-8493-7649-1
Library of Congress Card Number 94-26483
Printed in the United States of America 1 2 3 4 5 6 7 8 9 0
Printed on acid-free paper

PREFACE

Heparin and low molecular weight heparins are the drugs of choice to prevent and treat both arterial and venous thrombosis. The principal rationale for their use is that heparin (and heparin-like compounds) accelerate the inhibition of coagulation enzymes (primarily thrombin) by their endogenous plasma inhibitor, antithrombin III. However, it has become increasingly apparent that heparin and low molecular weight heparins do not always work as well as it was initially thought and hoped. Moreover, heparin has a number of significant side-effects, including bleeding and heparin-induced thrombocytopenia. A number of studies in the 1980's and earlier have increased our understanding of how thrombin interacts with its substrates, cofactors and endogenous inhibitors, and how thrombin alters the normal thromboresistance of the vessel wall after injury, contributing to thrombus formation and growth. How thrombin regulates its overproduction by activating circulating cells and other plasma cofactors and zymogens is also better appreciated. These recent studies have given us a better understanding of the limitations of heparin. An important observation made in these studies is that thrombin becomes resistant to inhibition by antithrombin III/heparin when the enzyme binds to a surface, be it to fibrin within a formed thrombus or to exposed components of a damaged vessel wall. This observation has been an important contributory factor in the efforts to develop other "anti-thrombins" which are able to inhibit thrombin by antithrombin III-independent mechanisms. These anti-thrombins include hirudin and a variety of synthetic peptides which inactivate thrombin directly, and other naturally occurring heparin-like catalysts such as dermatan sulfate, which accelerate the inhibition of thrombin by another of its endogenous inhibitors in plasma, heparin cofactor II, even when thrombin is bound to surfaces.

This book provides an indepth review of many of these recent studies, focusing on the roles of thrombin in venous and arterial thrombosis, its roles in regulating coagulation, the interactions of the enzyme with its endogenous inhibitors, and the relative effectiveness of antithrombin III-dependent, antithrombin III-independent and direct thrombin inhibitors in regulating the enzymatic activities of thrombin.

In Chapter 1, Ofosu et al. describe how thrombin accelerates and decelerates coagulation. Chapter 2 by Bode and Stubbs describes how visualizing the X-ray structures of thrombin have helped to better define the interactions of thrombin with its substrates and inhibitors. With this basic information background, Leclerc reviews the development and rationale for using low molecular weight heparins to prevent and treat venous thrombosis in Chapter 3. Buchanan et al.

then discuss the emerging concept for a potential role of heparin cofactor II catalysis (by dermatan sulfate) in the prevention and treatment of thrombosis (Chapter 4). A better understanding of the role of thrombin in thrombin generation and thrombus formation, and the benefits and limitations of heparin and low molecular weight heparins have justified the development and use of alternate thrombin inhibitors to prevent and treat arterial and venous thrombosis. Ginsberg reviews these issues in Chapter 5. Brister et al. then review the development and rationale for using other anti-thrombins to prevent and treat arterial thrombosis (Chapter 6). In Chapter 7, Andrew and David extensively review the differences in pediatric and adult coagulation, and how these differences influence the etiology of thrombosis and the implementation of strategies for preventing and treating thrombosis in these two populations. In Chapter 8, Prins reviews the role of thrombin inhibitors in thrombolytic therapy. Ginsberg and Brill-Edwards examine the hemostatic system in pregnancy, how thrombosis in pregnancy is influenced by altered thrombin generation, and how enhancing thrombin inhibition can ameliorate thrombosis in pregnancy (Chapter 9). Falanga, Cortelazzo and Barbui review the role of thrombin in thrombogenesis associated with metastasis (Chapter 10).

In summary, some chapters provide an extensive review of the current knowledge on which current antithrombotic/anticoagulant treatments are based. Other chapters review the newer concepts in managing thromboembolism and also identify unresolved issues.

THE EDITORS

Michael R. Buchanan, PhD, is a Professor of Department of Pathology, McMaster University, a Senior Scientist at the Hamilton Civic Hospitals Research Center and the Director of Surgical Research at the Hamilton Civic Hospitals, Hamilton, Ontario.

Dr. Buchanan completed his undergraduate studies at the University of Toronto in 1970 and then obtained his MSc and PhD in Medical Sciences at McMaster University in 1974 and 1978. He was also a Research Fellow in the Department of Pathology at Harvard University and a Research Associate at the Peter Bent Brigham Hospital, Boston, Massachusetts.

Dr. Buchanan is a member of the International Society of Thrombosis and Haemostasis, the American Heart Association, Council on Thrombosis, the Canadian Atherosclerosis Society, the International Society of Applied Cardiovascular Biology, the New York Academy of Sciences, the Canadian Cardiovascular Society and the Royal Society of Medicine.

Among other awards, Dr. Buchanan has received a number of Career Investigator Awards from the Canadian Heart Foundation and was the recipient of the 3rd Sanofi Foundation for Thrombosis Research prize, awarded at the International Society of Thrombosis and Haemostasis meeting in Tokyo in 1989.

Dr. Buchanan has presented many invited lectures at various universities, institutions and international meetings. He has also published over 200 research papers which address his current interests of basic and applied studies investigating 1) fatty acid metabolism as it relates to integrin expression by circulating blood and vessel wall cells, and their subsequent effects on thrombosis and metastasis; and 2) the relative effects of various anticoagulants including dermatan sulfate on the inhibition of circulating versus bound thrombin, and their subsequent benefits in venous and arterial thrombosis.

Stephanie J. Brister, MD, FRCS, is a Cardiovascular Surgeon at the Hamilton Civic Hospitals, Hamilton General Division, an Associate Member of the Hamilton Civic Hospitals Research Center, and an Associate Clinical Professor with McMaster University.

Dr. Brister completed her undergraduate studies at the University of Calgary in Biology in 1975 and obtained her MD degree from the University of Calgary in 1979. She subsequently trained in General Surgery at McGill University in Montreal, in Cardiovascular and Thoracic Surgery at Queen's University, followed by a Clinical Fellowship at the University of Toronto. In 1989, she set up a clinical practice in Hamilton. In addition, Dr. Brister set up a pulmonary thromboendarterectomy surgical program at the Hamilton General Hospital, and began studies with Drs. Ofosu and Buchanan in anticoagulant research as it relates to cardiovascular surgery. She has presented over 40 abstracts at national and international meetings and published a number of papers in this area.

Dr. Brister is currently a Fellow of the Royal College of Surgeons in Canada and a member of the Canadian Cardiovascular Society. In addition to her clinical interests, Dr. Brister's current research interests include investigating the relative effects of anticoagulants on the inhibition of circulating versus bound thrombin as it relates to achieving benefits in cardiac surgery while ameliorating bleeding and other adverse side-effects.

Dr. Frederick A. Ofosu, PhD, is a Professor in the Department of Pathology, McMaster University, Hamilton, Ontario and Senior Scientist, The Canadian Red Cross Society, Blood Services, in Hamilton, Ontario. Dr. Ofosu completed his undergraduate studies in Biochemistry at McMaster University (BSc, 1967), completed his graduate studies in Biochemistry at the University of Toronto (PhD, 1971) and spent his Research Fellowship at the Hospital for Sick Children, Toronto, Ontario.

Dr. Ofosu is a member of the International Society of Thrombosis and Haemostasis, Council of Thrombosis, American Heart Association, The Biochemical Society, Canadian Atherosclerosis Society, Canadian Society of Biochemistry and Molecular Biology. He was a member of the Sub-Committees on Heparin, Factor VIII and Factor IX, International Committee of Thrombosis and Haemostasis.

He is currently a member of the Expert Advisory Panel, Health Laboratory Services, the World Health Organization, Geneva, Switzerland. He organized the highly successful New York Academy of Sciences International Symposium on Heparin and Related Polysaccharides in 1987. His research is focused on the mechanisms of action of anticoagulant and antithrombotic drugs, areas he and his collaborators have made significant contributions during the past 10 years. He is invited regularly to present at major European meetings addressing issues on Thrombosis and Haemostasis.

CONTRIBUTORS

Maureen Andrew, MD
Department Pediatrics
Hamilton Civic Hospitals
Research Centre
Henderson Division
711 Concession St
Hamilton, Ontario
Canada

Tiziano Barbui, MD
Department Hematology
Ospedali Riuniti
Largo Barozzi, 1
24100 Bergamo
Italy

Enrico Bernardi, MD
Department Internal Medicine
University of Padua
Padua
Italy

Wolfram Bode, Dr.rer.nat
Max-Planck-Institut Fur Biochimic
82152 Martinsreid bei Munchei
Germany

Stephanie Brister, MD, FRCS(C)
Department Surgery
293 Wellington St N, Suite 132
Hamilton, Ontario
Canada

Michael Buchanan, PhD
Department Surgical Research
Hamilton Civic Hospitals
General Division
237 Barton St East, Room 418
Hamilton, Ontario
Canada

Sergio Cortelazzo, MD
Department of Hematology
Ospedali Riuniti
Largo Barozzi, 1
24100 Bergamo
Italy

Michele David, MD
Hopital Ste Justine
3175 Cote Ste-Catharine
Montreal, Quebec
Canada

Patrick Brill-Edwards, MD, FRCP(C), FACP
Department Medicine
McMaster University Health Sciences Centre
1200 Main St West, HSC-3W12
Hamilton, Ontario
Canada

Anna Falanga, MD
Department Hematology
Ospedali Riuniti
Largo Barozzi, 1
Italy

Jeffrey Ginsberg, MD, FRCP(C)
Department of Medicine
McMaster University Health
Sciences Centre
1200 Main St West, HSC-3W15
Hamilton, Ontario
Canada

Bruno Girolami, MD
Department Internal Medicine
University of Padua
Padua
Italy

Frederick Ofosu, PhD
Department Pathology
McMaster University Health
Sciences Centre
1200 Main St West, HSC-3N10
Hamilton, Ontario
Canada

Martin Prins, MD, PhD
Department Clin Epidemiology
Academic Med Centre B2-246
Meibergdreg g 1051 A2
Amsterdam
The Netherlands

Milton T. Stubbs, D.Phil
Max-Planck-Institut Fur Biochimic
82152 Martinsreid bei Munchei
Germany

ACKNOWLEDGEMENTS

Thanks to Dianne Walker for her secretarial assistance and a special thanks to Rachel Swaney for rendering this book in its final "camera ready" format.

TABLE OF CONTENTS

Chapter 3
DEVELOPMENT AND RATIONALE FOR THE USE OF LOW MOLECULAR WEIGHT HEPARINS IN THE PREVENTION AND TREATMENT OF VENOUS THROMBOSIS
Jacques R. Leclerc

Chapter 4

HEPARIN COFACTOR II AND THE PREVENTION AND TREATMENT OF THROMBOSIS

Michael R. Buchanan, Stephanie J. Brister and Frederick A. Ofosu

Chapter 5

DEVELOPMENT AND RATIONALE FOR THE USE OF DIRECT THROMBIN INHIBITORS IN THE PREVENTION AND TREATMENT OF ARTERIAL AND VENOUS THROMBOSIS

Jeffrey S. Ginsberg

Chapter 6
DEVELOPMENT AND RATIONALE FOR USE OF ANTI-THROMBINS IN ARTERIAL THROMBOSIS
Stephanie J. Brister, Frederick A. Ofosu and Michael R. Buchanan

Chapter 7
PEDIATRIC THROMBOEMBOLISM: EPIDEMIOLOGY, PREVENTION AND TREATMENT
Maureen Andrew and Michèle David

Chapter 1

THROMBIN-CATALYZED AMPLIFICATION AND INHIBITORY REACTIONS OF BLOOD COAGULATION

Frederick A. Ofosu, Michael R. Buchanan and Stephanie J. Brister

I. INTRODUCTION

Thrombin plays a central role in thrombogenesis because it is the only procoagulant enzyme capable of cleaving fibrinogen to fibrin, thereby initiating solid clot formation. It is essential, however, that thrombin generation and activity are regulated in such a manner that it proceeds only to an extent necessary for hemostasis. In this chapter, we review the reactions and interactions of (pro)thrombin with other blood components which orchestrate clot formation in a regulated manner, focusing on the reactions of α-thrombin, which accelerates and decelerates coagulation.

II. ACCELERATION OF BLOOD COAGULATION

α-Thrombin is the most active form of thrombin. It catalyzes three groups of reactions which regulate the propagation of blood coagulation. The first group of reactions involves cell activation to provide coagulant surfaces on which the enzyme complex prothrombinase assembles. Prothrombinase is the physiologic activator of prothrombin and consists of equimolar concentrations of the enzyme Factor Xa and its cofactor Factor Va bound to coagulant surfaces in the presence of ionic calcium.[1-3] This enzyme complex converts prothrombin into equimolar α-thrombin and prothrombin fragment 1+2 (F1+2). Because thrombin is rapidly inactivated by its endogenous plasma inhibitors, the concentration of prothrombin F1+2 in plasma is used to estimate thrombin production *in vivo* and *in vitro*.[4,5] The second group of thrombin-catalyzed reactions provides the cofactors, Factor Va and Factor VIIIa, and the enzyme, Factor XIa, all necessary for propagation of coagulation, and Factor XIIIa, the fibrin stabilizing enzyme. The third group of α-thrombin-dependent reactions provides the means for inactivating Factor Va and Factor VIIIa to suppress the propagation of blood coagulation.

The current concepts about the key reactions of the blood coagulation scheme, emphasizing the three reactions α-thrombin catalyses to accelerate the penultimate reaction of blood coagulation,

0-8493-7649-1/95/$0.00+$.50

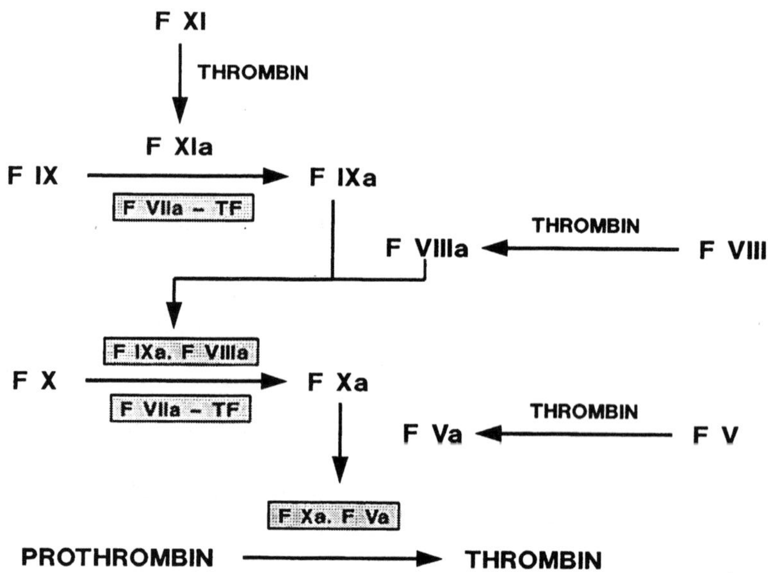

Figure 1. Direct actions of α-thrombin which accelerate prothrombinase formation. Thrombin-mediated activation of Factor XI accelerates Factor IX activation. Activation of Factor VIII and Factor V by thrombin accelerates intrinsic tenase (Factor IXa-Factor VIIIa) and prothrombinase (Factor Xa-Factor Va) formation, respectively. The three membrane-bound enzyme complexes are enclosed in shaded rectangles.

namely, the assembly of prothrombinase are summarized in Fig. 1. The final reactions of coagulation are the conversion of soluble fibrinogen to insoluble fibrin by α-thrombin and the stabilization of fibrin by Factor XIIIa (not shown in Fig. 1). α-Thrombin cleaves two peptides, fibrinopeptide A and B, from fibrinogen to initiate the polymerization of fibrin.[3] The coagulation reactions are essentially a series of limited proteolytic reactions catalyzed by serine proteases which usually require cofactors and surfaces to optimize their proteolytic activities.[1-4] The appropriate cofactors and coagulant surfaces increase the catalytic efficiency of the reactions in question by several orders of magnitude.[2] The protein cofactors of coagulation are tissue Factor (for Factor VIIa), Factor Va (for Factor Xa), and Factor VIIIa (for Factor IXa), endothelial cell surface thrombomodulin (for α-thrombin when it activates protein C), fibrin (for α-thrombin when it activates Factor XIII) and the vitamin K-dependent clotting Factor protein S (for activated protein C). Ionic calcium is also required for all of the coagulation reactions which require surfaces and cofactors. The interactions of α-thrombin with cells which provide cell surfaces for assembling the enzyme complexes of blood coagulation, the reactions of α-thrombin which provide Factor Va and Factor VIIIa, and the reactions of α-thrombin which decelerate coagulation are discussed separately below.

A. EXPRESSION OF COAGULANT SURFACES

The Factor VIIa-tissue Factor (extrinsic tenase and extrinsic ninease, namely, Factor X and Factor IX activators during extrinsic coagulation), the Factor IXa-Factor VIIIa (intrinsic tenase or Factor X activator during intrinsic coagulation) and the Factor Xa-Factor Va (prothrombinase) enzyme complexes must be assembled on coagulant surfaces to express their full enzymatic activities.[1-4] Essentially, all blood-borne cells and endothelial cells can support prothrombinase assembly.[6,7] While coagulant phospholipids (L-α-phosphatidylcholine and L-α-phosphatidylserine in a ratio of ~70:30) will optimally support the assembly of the three enzyme complexes *in vitro*[8], they are likely to be assembled on intact cells *in vivo*. For example, tissue Factor, the cofactor for the enzyme Factor VIIa, is expressed constitutively at very low levels on monocytes[7] and on smooth muscle cells[9], and can become expressed on activated endothelial cells.[10] Activated platelets likely provide the principal surfaces on which intrinsic tenase and prothrombinase assemble *in vivo*[2,4], although peripheral blood mononuclear cells (lymphocyte, monocyte, and macrophages), smooth muscle cells, and endothelial cells also support the assembly of tenases and prothrombinase *in vitro*[6,7,9,10] and may also do so *in vivo*. α-Thrombin is the most potent physiologic activator of platelets. Approximately 1.0 nM α-thrombin can bind platelets to initiate the activation of platelets suspended in plasma[11], and sub-nanomolar concentrations of α-thrombin can bind and activate washed platelets.[12-14] The requirement for higher concentrations of α-thrombin for activating platelets in plasma likely reflects a competition between platelets and other α-thrombin substrates and inhibitors in plasma. α-Thrombin-mediated platelet activation precedes the assembly of platelet-bound prothrombinase in platelet-rich plasma.[11] α-Thrombin also binds endothelial cells, smooth muscle cells and mononuclear cells in a manner analogous to its binding to platelets.[15-17] However, whether and how α-thrombin activates endothelial cells, smooth muscle cells, and leukocytes to accelerate the assembly of prothrombinase on the surface of these cells have yet to be established.

α-Thrombin activates platelets by cleaving off a 41-mer peptide from the amino terminal extracellular domain of one of the two reported receptors of α-thrombin on platelets, a member of the seven-transmembrane G-protein-coupled receptor family.[18] The second reported α-thrombin receptor on platelets is the integrin GPIb.[19] How α-thrombin interacts with GPIb to activate platelets has not yet been defined. A few residues downstream from the α-thrombin cleavage site of the seven transmembrane α-thrombin receptor on platelets is a hirudin tail-like domain to which α-thrombin binds.[13,20] Cleavage and release of the 41-mer activation peptide from platelets is accompanied by transmission of secondary messages within the platelets, with the resultant secretion of constituents from platelet storage granules.[11,18,21,22] When α-thrombin is added to recalcified platelet-rich plasma (which also contains 1 μM tick anticoagulant peptide, a Factor Xa inhibitor [23], at a concentration that abrogates endogenous α-thrombin production in the platelet-rich plasma), the enzyme binds to the platelets in a concentration-dependent manner. α-Thrombin binding to the platelets and the subsequent platelet activation both proceed to completion within 10 seconds. A monoclonal antibody to part of the hirudin tail-like region of the receptor[13] abrogates thrombin binding to and activation of platelets suspended in plasma.[24] Thus, this member of the seven-transmembrane receptor family is an important site where α-thrombin binds to platelets in their natural medium (i.e. plasma). As noted previously, this receptor is also found on endothelial cells, smooth muscle cells and leukocytes, and α-thrombin also binds to these cells via the same receptor. Whether cleavage and release of the 41-mer activation peptide from endothelial cells and smooth muscle cells necessarily leads to their "activation" in a manner analogous to that of platelets has yet to be established.

In any event, cleavage of this 41-mer activation peptide from platelets by α-thrombin precedes the assembly of platelet-bound prothrombinase in platelet-rich plasma. Specifically, when platelet-rich plasma is recalcified, binding of endogenous α-thrombin to the platelets and the resulting release from platelets storage granules (measured as the appearance of P-selectin (GMP-140) on the platelet membrane surface) begin when the concentration of prothrombin F1+2 generated in the platelet-rich plasma increases by ~1 nM and proceeds to completion a few seconds later. These events are followed 2 to 5 minutes later by rapid and efficient prothrombin activation.[20] However, maximum α-thrombin binding to the platelets, the associated platelet activation and secretion of platelet granule contents may not provide the necessary and sufficient conditions for optimizing prothrombinase assembly. Additional but undefined changes in the platelet surface may be required before the activated platelets will fully support prothrombinase assembly. When α-thrombin is added to platelet-rich plasma, both α-thrombin binding to platelets and the subsequent platelet activation proceed to completion within 10 seconds. In addition to activating the platelets, the α-thrombin also activates Factor V in the plasma. If cleavage of the thrombin receptor and the associated platelet secretion necessarily support optimal prothrombinase assembly, it is reasonable to expect prothrombin activation to proceed as rapidly and efficiently as it does in platelet-poor plasma which has been pre-incubated with 10 nM α-thrombin, and then supplemented with coagulant phospho- lipids and Factor Xa. Factor Xa is the only missing constituent for platelet-bound prothrombinase assembly since the platelet-rich plasma already contains Factor Va. Compared to the platelet-poor plasma, however, prothrombin activation initially proceeds rather slowly after Factor Xa is added to platelet-rich plasma pre-incubated with α-thrombin and $CaCl_2$ for exactly 10 seconds.

B. ACTIVATION OF FACTOR V AND FACTOR VIII

Factor Va light and heavy chains constitute Factor Va, the cofactor required for prothrombin activation by Factor Xa.[1-3] Two fragments derived from Factor VIII heavy chain and a third fragment derived from Factor VIII light chain constitute Factor VIIIa, the cofactor for Factor X activation by Factor IXa.[2,25] Factor Va and Factor VIIIa accelerate prothrombin and Factor X activation, respectively, by several orders of magnitude.[1,2] The concentrations of Factor Va and Factor VIIIa in plasma will, therefore, essentially regulate the rates of prothrombin and Factor X activation, respectively. Factor Xa and thrombin activate purified Factor V with similar catalytic efficiency.[26] Therefore, both enzymes have the potential to activate Factor V during plasma coagulation. Activation of Factor V by α-thrombin and Factor Xa during coagulation have been investigated by comparing the inhibition of prothrombin activation by dermatan sulfate and a synthetic pentasaccharide with high affinity for antithrombin III (ATIII) in contact-activated plasma. The pentasaccharide only catalyzes Factor Xa inhibition by ATIII[27], while dermatan sulfate only catalyzes thrombin inhibition by heparin cofactor II (HCII).[28] On a mole-for-mole basis, dermatan sulfate is tenfold more effective in delaying the initiation of prothrombin activation than the pentasaccharide.[29] Thus, during prothrombin activation in plasma, endogenous α-thrombin appears to activate Factor V more effectively than endogenous Factor Xa.

As noted below, sub-nanomolar prothrombinase can effectively activate plasma prothrombin, compared to the micromolar concentrations of dermatan sulfate and the pentasaccharide required to delay the initiation of intrinsic prothrombin activation[29], i.e. to inhibit the formation of sub-nanomolar prothrombinase. Therefore, hirudin, a direct and more potent α-thrombin inhibitor than dermatan sulfate, was added to plasmas in order to re-assess the roles of Factor Xa and thrombin plasma Factor V activators. Factor X-depleted plasma was also the plasma used for this comparison since it does not generate Factor Xa, making it a more suitable plasma than normal plasma for defining the minimum concentration of Factor Xa that can activate plasma Factor V. Hirudin was used to inactivate thrombin as it was produced in the plasma to determine the contribution of endogenous thrombin to Factor V activation during plasma coagulant. When prothrombin activation is initiated by adding a suspension containing Factor Xa, $CaCl_2$, and coagulant phospholipids to the Factor X-depleted plasma, the only requirement for prothrombinase assembly is Factor Va, in turn generated *in situ* by the exogenous Factor Xa and/or endogenous α-thrombin. Prothrombin activation begins without a lag phase with 0.5 nM Factor Xa, and proceeds to completion within ~100 seconds of its initiation (Fig. 2). The initiation of prothrombin activation is delayed by 10 nM, which then continues to suppress prothrombin activation when it begins. A tenfold higher concentraton hirudin abrogates prothrombin activation. When the concentration of Factor Xa is increased to 1.0 nM, 1 μM hirudin also abrogates prothrombin activation (not shown). However, when the concentration of Factor Xa is increased to 5 nM, even 100 μM hirudin cannot abrogate prothrombin activation. Thus, ~5 nM Factor Va can initiate plasma Factor V activation to facilitate prothrombinase assembly. However, endogenous α-thrombin also contributes to Factor V activation to optimize prothrombinase assembly in this plasma. If the Factor X-depleted plasma is pretreated with 0.5, 1.0 or 5.0 nM α-thrombin for only 10 seconds before introducing 0.5 nM Factor Xa, Ca^{2+}, and coagulant phospholipids, even 100 μM hirudin no longer abrogates prothrombin activation (not shown). These effects of hirudin suggest that α-thrombin activates plasma Factor V more efficiently than Factor Xa, and that even when 5 nM Factor Xa initiates Factor V activation in plasma, the α-thrombin formed therein also activates Factor V to optimize prothrombinase formation.

α-Thrombin is probably the only enzyme that activates Factor VIII in plasma, where Factor VIII is complexed to its carrier protein, von Willebrand Factor.[30,31] Factor VIII bound to von Willebrand Factor is not activated by Factor Xa.[30,31] Thrombin activates Factor VIII by cleaving the protein after Arg 372, Arg 740, and Arg 1689.[25,31] Two fragments derived from Factor VIII heavy chain, apparent Mr 50 and 43 kDa, and a light chain fragment, apparent Mr 73 kDa, constitute Factor VIIIa. α-Thrombin also inactivates Factor VIIIa[25,31], with α-thrombin being ~100-fold more efficient than Factor Xa or activated protein C.[31] α-Thrombin inactivates Factor VIIIa by cleaving the 43 kDa heavy chain-derived fragment after Arg 562. Both Factor Xa and activated protein C inactivate Factor VIIIa by cleaving the 50 kDa fragment after Arg 336 into a 45 kDa fragment.[25,31] Thus, thrombin

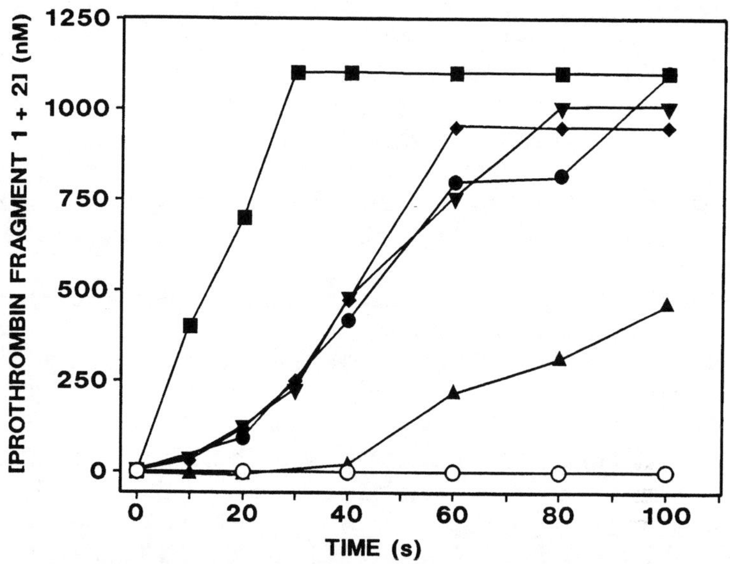

Figure 2. Use of hirudin to estimate plasma Factor V activation by Factor Xa and α-thrombin. Arvin-defibrinated Factor X-depleted plasma, with and without hirudin, was pre-warmed to 37°C and incubated with an equal volume of a coagulant suspension containing Factor Xa, $CaCl_2$ and platelin. Prothrombin activation was then quantified as prothrombin fragment 1+2 production. Increasing concentrations of hirudin were added to the plasma to inactivate thrombin as it was formed. Symbols: ●, 0.5 nM Factor Xa; ▲, 0.5 nM Factor Xa + 10 nM hirudin; o, 0.5 nM Factor Xa + 100 nM hirudin; ■, 5 nM Factor Xa; ♦, 5 nM Factor Xa + 10 μM hirudin; ▼, 5 nM Factor Xa + 100 μM hirudin.

both activates Factor VIII and inactivates Factor VIIIa to regulate its own production.

C. ACTIVATION OF FACTOR XIII

Factor XIIIa is a transamidase which cross-links fibrin by forming amide bonds involving the γ-carboxylate groups of glutamate and the ε-amino groups of lysine, forming Nε-(γ-glutamyl) lysine bonds.[3,32] Cross-linking of fibrin by Factor XIIIa stabilizes clots since the fibrin becomes less resistant to lysis by plasmin. α-Thrombin-mediated activation of Factor XIII requires ionic calcium and is markedly enhanced by fibrin.[3,32] As noted above, α-thrombin converts fibrinogen into fibrin I by cleaving fibrinopeptide A from fibrinogen. It converts fibrinogen and fibrin I into fibrin II by cleaving of both fibrinopeptides A and B, from fibrinogen and fibrinopeptide B from fibrin I.[3] Fibrinopeptide A release is the minimum required to initiate the initial and non-covalent polymerization of fibrin. α-Thrombin associates non-covalently with both fibrin I and fibrin II, where the reactivity of the enzyme with small molecular weight substrates essentially remains unchanged.[33,34] The site on α-thrombin to which fibrin binds, known as the fibrin(ogen) recognition exosite, is also where the enzyme binds to thrombomodulin, plate- lets, ATIII, and hirudin.[35,37] Although there may be additional sites on α-thrombin to which fibrin and the other four agents also bind, the fibrin(ogen) recognition exosite is the site on α-thrombin to which thrombomodulin, platelets, fibrinogen, ATIII and hirudin initially bind the enzyme.[35,37]

As noted above, the association of α-thrombin with fibrin accelerates Factor XIII activation by α-thrombin. Fibrin I similarly accelerates intrinsic prothrombin and Factor X activation. Fibrin I also accelerates Factor X and prothrombin activation when a suspension containing α-thrombin, $CaCl_2$ and coagulant phospholipids is added to plasma.[38] Thus, it is likely that fibrin decreases the specific cleavage which leads to the inactivation of the cofactor of Factor VIIIa by α-thrombin. There is no direct evidence to support this idea, however. Fibrin modulates other reactions of α-thrombin; for example, fibrin I and II decrease the reactivity of α-thrombin with ATIII, both in the presence and absence of heparin.[39,40] It is noteworthy that fibrin does not moderate the inactivation of thrombin by HCII or dermatan sulfate-HCII.[38]

D. FACTOR XI ACTIVATION

Two groups have reported independently α-thrombin-mediated activation of purified Factor XI.[5,41] One of the groups has subsequently reported thrombin also contributes to Factor XI activation in plasma to which diluted tissue Factor was added.[42] The significance of these observations is that where tissue Factor expression is limited (as is likely to be the case most of the time *in vivo*), propagation of coagulation probably requires Factor IX activation by Factor XIa to sustain Factor X activation by intrinsic tenase (the Factor IXa-Factor VIIIa enzyme complex). Activation of Factor IX by Factor XIa *in vivo* would be particularly critical if Factor VIIa-tissue Factor is rapidly inactivated by tissue Factor pathway inhibitor when Factor Xa also becomes available. A quaternary complex containing equimolar tissue Factor, Factor VIIa, tissue Factor pathway inhibitor, and Factor Xa is formed in the presence of Ca^{2+}.[43] Neither Factor VIIa nor Factor Xa within this quaternary complex retains its enzymatic activity. Thus, unless Factor VIIa-tissue Factor can activate Factor IX as efficiently as Factor X, Factor XIa availability would be essential to propagate coagulation initiated by Factor VIIa-tissue Factor.

E. THROMBIN-DEPENDENT ANTICOAGULANT REACTIONS

As noted previously, Factor Va and Factor VIIIa increase the rates of prothrombin and Factor X activation by several orders of magnitude, respectively, and α-thrombin activates both Factor V and Factor VIII. Therefore, two broad approaches for reducing the rates of Factor X and prothrombin activation in plasma are 1) enhancing the intrinsic capacity of plasma to inactivate thrombin to decrease α-thrombin-mediated activation of Factor V and Factor VIII, and 2) inactivating both Factor Va and Factor VIIIa directly. Two of α-thrombin inhibitors endogenous to plasma are ATIII and HCII. Heparin catalyzes α-thrombin inhibition by ATIII whereas dermatan sulfate catalyzes α-thrombin inhibition by HCII.[28,44] Enhancing endogenous α-thrombin inhibition by catalysts, or by a direct α-thrombin inhibitor, such as hirudin, decreases the availability of Factor Va and Factor VIIIa in plasma[44-46] (see also Chapters 4, 5, 6, 7, and 8 for additional discussion on strategies for enhancing thrombin inhibition in plasma). Limited proteolysis of Factor VIIIa by α-thrombin and Factor Xa, and limited proteolysis of Factor Va and Factor VIIIa by activated protein C are the only known direct means for inactivating plasma Factor Va and Factor VIIIa.[25,31,47] The direct and indirect actions of α-thrombin which inactivate Factor Va and Factor VIIIa are summarized in Fig. 3.

As noted above, α-thrombin both activates Factor VIII and inactivates Factor VIIIa by limited proteolysis (Figs. 1 and 3). Factor Xa and activated protein C also inactivate Factor VIIIa.[25,31] When equimolar concentrations of the three enzymes are compared, thrombin inactivates Factor VIIIa 100 times more effectively than Factor Xa or activated protein C.[31] Thrombin also activates protein C by limited proteolysis, in a reaction enhanced ~1000-fold by endothelial cell-associated thrombomodulin.[47] Thrombomodulin forms a 1:1 complex with α-thrombin (K_d ~1.0 nM) by binding α-thrombin at the fibrin(ogen) recognition exosite, the site with which the enzyme interacts with ATIII, fibrin and platelets. It is possible, therefore, for fibrin(ogen), platelets and ATIII to decrease the complexation of thrombin with thrombomodulin *in vivo*. How effectively these potential antagonists of thrombomodulin influence the binding of α-thrombin to thrombomodulin will depend largely on the concentrations of fibrinogen, endothelial cell thrombomodulin, endothelial cell and platelet receptors for α-thrombin at site of α-thrombin production *in vivo*, and their affinities for α-thrombin.

Notwithstanding the foregoing, thrombomodulin has the potential to inhibit the propagation of coagulation by two mechanisms, namely, 1) direct inhibition of α-thrombin-mediated activation of Factor V and Factor VIII, and 2) acceleration of protein C activation by α-thrombin (Fig. 3). Thrombomodulin competitively inhibits α-thrombin-mediated proteolysis of fibrinogen and Factor V.[48] Whether thrombomodulin also competitively inhibits thrombin-mediated Factor VIII activation and

1. FACTOR VIIIa —THROMBIN→ FACTOR VIIIi

2. PROTEIN C —THROMBIN–TM→ ACTIVATED PROTEIN C

3. FACTOR VIIIa —APC→ FACTOR VIIIi

4. FACTOR Va —APC→ FACTOR Vi

Figure 3. Direct and indirect actions of α-thrombin which inhibit prothrombinase formation and inactivate prothrombinase. α-Thrombin cleaves Factor VIIIa into inactive Factor VIIIa (Factor VIIIi). α-Thrombin binds thrombomodulin to activate protein C. Activated protein C (APC), in turn, proteolyses Factor VIIIa and Factor Va into the inactivate products Factor VIIIi and Factor Vi, respectively. Note that APC and α-thrombin inactivate Factor VIIIa by cleaving two different peptide bonds in Factor VIIIa.

inactivation of Factor VIIIa has not been reported. The extent to which thrombomodulin directly (and thus competitively) inhibits plasma prothrombinase assembly is also not well established. Whether thrombin-thrombomodulin catalyzes plasma protein C activation to the extent necessary for the activated protein C generated to influence prothrombinase formation, or to inactivate prothrombinase, has similarly not been determined. It is important to recognize that the concentration of plasma prothrombinase that converts essentially all prothrombin into thrombin and prothrombin F1+2 within 120 seconds of initiating plasma prothrombin activation is less than 1 nM (see Figs. 2 and 4). Thus, in order for thrombomodulin to abrogate prothrombin activation, both competitive inhibition of α-thrombin-mediated Factor VIII and Factor V activation and the enhancement of α-thrombin-mediated protein C activation by thrombomodulin must be rapid enough to abrogate the incorporation of Factor Va into prothrombinase.

Suppression of plasma prothrombin activation by recombinant (r-) human thrombomodulin, r-human activated protein C, and hirudin have been compared in recent experiments. Hirudin is the most potent known inhibitor of α-thrombin[49] and equimolar hirudin abrogates α-thrombin-mediated activation of Factor V in plasma.[46] Therefore, hirudin probably provides the best means for estimating the extent to which effective inhibition of endogenous α-thrombin can

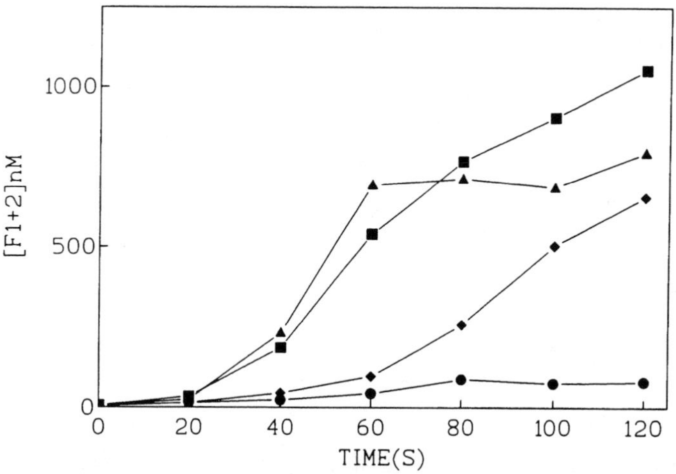

Figure 4. Inhibition of prothrombin activation by hirudin, thrombomodulin and activated protein C. Prothrombin activation was initiated by adding a suspension containing 1.0 nM Factor Xa, 20 mM $CaCl_2$ and platelin to an equal volume of Factor X-depleted plasma (■); Factor X-depleted plasma containing 20 nM hirudin (♦); Factor X-depleted plasma containing 20 nM r-human thrombomodulin (▲), or Factor X-depleted plasma containing 20nM r-activated protein C (●). Prothrombin activation was quantified as prothrombin fragment 1+2 production.

inhibit prothrombinase assembly. Each inhibitor was used at a concentration of 10 nM in plasma, the minimum concentration of α-thrombin which activates all plasma Factor V within 60 seconds of adding the enzyme to plasma.[44,46] As summarized in Figs. 2 and 4, 10 nM hirudin delays the initiation of prothrombin activation in Factor X-depleted plasma supplemented with 0.5 nM Factor Xa, and also inhibits prothrombin activation after it begins. These effects of hirudin suggest that Factor Xa is rapidly inactivated in plasma until Factor Va becomes available and the enzyme then becomes incorporated into prothrombinase. Once incorporated into pro- thrombinase, the Factor Xa then becomes more difficult to inactivate by its natural inhibitors in plasma.

Like hirudin, activated protein C delays the initiation of prothrombin activation. In contrast to hirudin and activated protein C, thrombomodulin cannot delay the initiation of prothrombin activation initiated by adding Factor Xa to 0.5 nM Factor X-depleted plasma (Fig. 4). However, prothrombin activation essentially ceases when the incubation of plasma containing thrombomodulin exceeds 60 seconds. This weaker initial anticoagulant action of thrombo-modulin, compared to that of activated protein C, suggests that up to 10 nM α-thrombin-thrombomodulin does not efficiently activate protein C in the plasma until the incubation increases to ~60 seconds of

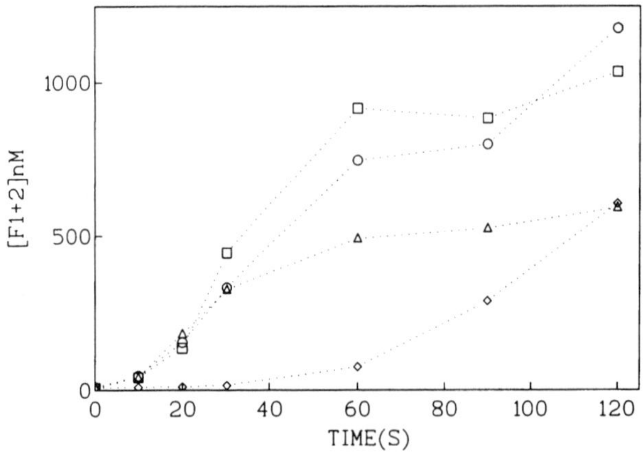

Figure 5. Effects of thrombomodulin and activated protein C on prothrombin activation in Factor X-depleted plasma containing Factor Va. Defibrinated Factor X-depleted plasma was incubated with 10 nM α-thrombin for 60 seconds to fully activate the Factor V. Following this, an equal volume of coagulant suspension containing 1 nM Factor Xa, 20 mM $CaCl_2$, and platelin was added to the plasma (□). In some experiments, the coagulant suspension also contained 20 nM activated protein C (○), or 20 nM thrombomodulin (△). In another experiment, the α-thrombin was added to Factor X-depleted plasma (◇) which already contained 10 nM hirudin to estimate how effectively it suppressed Factor V activation by the added α-thrombin.

incubation. Subsequently, enough activated protein C is produced to essentially prevent additional prothrombin activation.

Inactivation of prothrombinase by thrombomodulin and activated protein C have also been investigated. Prothrombinase is generated in Factor X-depleted plasma by pre-incubating it with 10 nM α-thrombin $CaCl_2$ and coagulant phospholipids for 60 seconds to activate the Factor V before Factor Xa is added to the plasma initiate prothrombin activation. Since Factor Xa is the enzyme and Factor Va is the cofactor of prothrombinase, hirudin, as expected, does not inactivate prothrombinase. As shown in Fig. 5, when the Factor X-depleted plasma already contains Factor Va before Factor Xa is added to it, prothrombin is activated more rapidly than in the control Factor X-depleted plasma (Fig. 2). During the first 20 seconds of incubation, prothrombin is activated at similar rates in the control and in the plasmas containing thrombomodulin or activated protein C. Subsequently, the rate of prothrombin activation decreases in the plasma containing thrombomodulin and activated protein C, but less so in the latter plasma (Fig. 5). Thus, it appears thrombomodulin inhibits prothrombin activation by similar actions in both plasmas, namely, by enhancing thrombin-mediated protein C activation. Activated protein C appears to inactivate Factor Va to prevent its incorporation into prothrombinase. However, it can achieve this action effectively only when the initial concentration of Factor Va is limited. Under the experimental conditions used, activated protein C does not appear to effectively inactivate Factor Va previously incorporated into prothrombinase.

III. SUMMARY

In addition to converting fibrinogen to fibrin to provide the primary protein component of blood clots, α-thrombin accelerates its own production by providing coagulant surfaces (by activating platelets), and two cofactors critical for thrombin production, namely, Factor Va and Factor VIIIa. α-Thrombin also activates Factor XI and thus indirectly increases the availability of Factor IXa (and thus, additional Factor Xa). The availability of Factor IXa provides the means for propagating coagulation once Factor VIIa-tissue Factor becomes inactivated within the quaternary tissue Factor-Factor VIIa-tissue Factor pathway inhibitor-Factor Xa complex. α-Thrombin also initiates fibrin stabilization by activating Factor XIII in the presence of fibrin and Ca^{2+}. In addition to these procoagulant actions, α-thrombin activates protein C (in the presence of thrombomodulin) to initiate two anti-coagulant actions. In the presence of thrombo-modulin, α-thrombin activates protein C, and activated protein C in turn, inactivates Factor Va (to inhibit prothrombin activation) and Factor VIIIa (to inhibit Factor X activation). In addition, α-thrombin inactivates Factor VIIIa to suppress Factor X activation by Factor IXa. What remains to be established is how the balance between the procoagulant and anti-coagulant functions of α-thrombin is achieved *in vivo*.

REFERENCES

1. **Davie, E.W., Fujikawa, K., Kisiel, W.** The coagulation cascade:initiation, maintainance and regulation. *Biochem* 30, 10363, 1991.
2. **Mann, K.G., Jenny, J.R., Krishnaswamy, S.** Cofactor proteins in the assembly and expression of blood clotting enzymes. *Ann Rev Biochem* 57, 915, 1988.
3. **Mann, K.G., Lorand, L.** Blood coagulation. *Methods Enzymol* 222, 1, 1993.
4. **Furie, B.C.** Molecular and cellular biology of blood coagulation. *N Engl J Med* 326, 800, 1992.
5. **Gailani, D., Broze, G.J., Jr.** Factor IX activation in revised model of blood coagulation. *Science* 253, 909, 1991.
6. **Tracy, P.B.** Regulation of thrombin generation at cell surfaces. *Semin Thromb Hemost* 14, 227, 1988.

7. **Tracy, P.B., Robinson, R.A., Worfolk, L.A., Allen, D.H.** Procoagulant activities expressed by peripheral blood mononuclear cells. *Methods Enzymol* 222, 281, 1993.
8. **Mann, K.G., Tracy, P.B., Krishnaswamy, S., Jenny, R.J., Odegaard, B.H., Nesheim, M.E.** Platelets and coagulation. In: *Thrombosis and Haemostasis*. M. Verstraete, J. Vermylen, R. Lijnen, J. Arnout (eds), Leuven University, Leuven, 1987, pp 505-523.
9. **Taubman, M.B., Marmur, J., Rosenfield, C-L, Guha, A., Nichtberger, S., Nemerson, Y.** Agonist-mediated tissue Factor expression in cultured vascular smooth muscle cells: Role of Ca^{2+} mobilization and protein kinase C activation. *J Clin Invest* 91, 547, 1993.
10. **Stern, D., Nawroth, P., Handley, D., Kisiel, W.** An endothelial cell-dependent pathway of coagulation. *Proc Natl Acad Sci USA* 82, 2523, 1985.
11. **Liu, L., Freedman, J., Hornstein, A., Dewar, L., Ofosu, F.A.** Effects of selective thrombin or Factor Xa inhibition on the assembly of platelet-bound prothrombinase in plasma. *Thromb Haemost* 69, 967, 1993.
12. **Harmon, J.T., Jamieson, G.A.** Activation of platelets by α-thrombin in a receptor mediated event. *J Biol Chem* 261, 15928, 1986.
13. **Brass, L.F., Vassallo, R.R., Jr., Belmonte, E., Ahuja, M., Cichowski, K., Hoxie, J.A.** Structure and function of the human platelet thrombin receptor. *J Biol Chem* 267, 13795, 1992.
14. **Norton, K.J., Scarborough, R.M., Kutok, J.L., Escobedo, M-A, Nannizzi, L., Coller, B.S.** Immunologic analysis of the cloned platelet thrombin receptor activation mechanism: Evidence supporting receptor cleavage, release of the N-terminal peptide, and insertion of the tethered ligand into a protected environment. *Blood* 82, 2125, 1993.
15. **Sugama, Y., Tirnppathi, C., Janakidevi, K., Andersen, T.T., Fenton, J.W., II, Malik, A.B.** Thrombin-induced expression of endothelial cell P-selectin and intracellular adhesion molecule-1: A mechanism for stabilizing neutrophil adhesion. *J Cell Biol* 119, 935, 1992.
16. **McNamara, C., Sarenbrok, I., Gimple, L.W., Fenton, J.W., II, Coughlin, S.R., Owens, G.K.** Thrombin stimulates proliferation of cultured rat aortic smooth muscle cells by a proteolytically activated receptor. *J Clin Invest* 91, 94, 1994.
17. **Zimmerman, G.P., McIntyre, T.M., Prescott, S.M.** Thrombin stimulates neutrophil adherence by an endothelial cell-dependent mechanism. *Ann NY Acad Sci* 485, 349, 1986.

18. **Vu, T-K.H., Hung, D.T., Wheaton, V.I., Coughlin, S.R.** Molecular cloning of a functional thrombin receptor reveals a novel proteolytic mechanism of receptor activation. *Cell* 64, 1057, 1991.
19. **Yamamoto, N., Greco, N.J., Barnard, M.R., Tanoue, K., Yamazaki, H., Jamieson, G.A., Michelson, A.D.** Glycoprotein (GPIb)-dependent and GPIb-independent pathways of thrombin-induced platelet activation. *Blood* 77, 1740, 1991.
20. **Liu, L., Vu, T-K, Esmon, C.T., Coughlin, S.** The region of the thrombin receptor resembling hirudin binds to thrombin and alters the enzyme specificity. *J Biol Chem* 266, 16977, 1991.
21. **Ishii, H., Hein, L., Kobilka, B., Coughlin, S.** Kinetics of thrombin receptor cleavage on intact cells relation to signalling. *J Biol Chem* 268, 9780, 1993.
22. **Vouret-Craviari, V., Van Obberghen-Schilling, E., Rasmussen, U.B., Pavirani, A., Lecocq, J-P, Pouyssegur, J.** Synthetic α-thrombin receptor peptides activate G protein coupled signalling pathways but are unable to induce mitogenesis. *Mol Cell Biol* 3, 95, 1992.
23. **Vlasuk, G.P.** Structural and functional characterization of tick anticoagulant peptide (TAP): A potent and selective inhibitor of blood coagulation Factor Xa. *Thromb Haemost* 70, 212, 1993.
24. **Liu, L., Freedman, J., Horstein, A., Fenton, J.W., II, Ofosu, F.A.** Thrombin binding to platelets and their activation in plasma. Submitted to *Br J Haematol*, 1994.
25. **Fay, P.J.** Factor VIII structure and function. *Thromb Haemost* 70, 63, 1993.
26. **Monkovic, D.D., Tracy, P.B.** Activation of human Factor V by Factor Xa and thrombin. *Biochem* 29, 1118, 1990.
27. **Choay, J.** Chemically synthesized heparin-derived oligosaccharides. *Ann NY Acad Sci* 556, 95, 1989.
28. **Tollefsen, D.M., Pestka, C.A., Monafo, W.J.** Activation of heparin cofactor II by dermatan sulfate. *J Biol Chem* 258, 6713, 1983.
29. **Ofosu, F.A., Choay, J., Anvari, N., Smith, L.M., Blajchman, M.A.** Inhibition of Factor X and Factor V activation by dermatan sulfate and the synthetic pentasaccharide with high affinity to antithrombin III. *Eur J Biochem* 193, 485, 1990.
30. **Koedman, J.A., Hamer, R.J., Beeser-Visser, N.H., Bouma, B.N., Sixma, J.J.** The effect of von Willebrand Factor on activation of Factor VIII by Factor Xa. *Eur J Biochem* 189, 229, 1990.
31. **Ying, L.** Identification of recombinant Factor VIII fragments generated by thrombin and Factor Xa using anti-Factor VIII peptide antibodies. M.Sc. Thesis, McMaster University, Hamilton, 1992.

32. **Lorand, L., Radek, J.T.** Activation of human plasma Factor XIII by thrombin in thrombin structure and function. In: *Thrombin Structure and Function*. L.J. Berliner (ed), Plenum Press, New York, 1992, pp 257-271.
33. **Liu, C.Y., Nossel, H.L., Kaplan, K.L.** The binding of thrombin by fibrin. *J Biol Chem* 254, 10421, 1979.
34. **Fenton, J.W., II, Ofosu, F.A., Breznick, D.V., Hassouna, H.I.** Understanding thrombin and hemostasis. *Hematol Oncol Clin North Am* 7, 1107, 1993.
35. **Grutter, M.G., Priestle, J.P., Rahuel, J., Grossenbacher, H., Bode, W., Hofsteenge, J., Stone, S.R.** Crystal structure of the thrombin-hirudin complex: a novel mode of serine protease inhibition. *EMBO J* 9, 2361, 1990.
36. **Rydel, T.J., Ravichandran, K.G., Tulinsky, A., Bode, W., Huber, R., Roitsch, C., Fenton, J.W., II.** The structure of a complex of recombinant hirudin and human α-thrombin. *Science* 249, 277, 1990.
37. **Stubbs, M.T., Oschkinat, H., Mayr, I., Huber, R., Angliker, H., Stone, S.R., Bode, W.** The interaction of thrombin with fibrinogen – a structural basis for its specificity. *Eur J Biochem* 206, 187, 1992.
38. **Okwusidi, J.I., Anvari, N., Ofosu, F.A.** Modulation of intrinsic prothrombin activation by fibrinogen and fibrin I. *J Lab Clin Med* 121, 64, 1993.
39. **Hogg, P.J., Jackson, C.M.** Fibrin monomer protects thrombin from inactivation by heparin-antithrombin III: Implications for heparin efficacy. *Proc Natl Acad Sci USA* 86, 3619, 1989.
40. **Okwusidi, J.I., Anvari, N., Kulczycky, M., Blajchman, M.A., Buchanan, M.R., Ofosu, F.A.** Fibrin moderates the catalytic activity of heparin but not that of dermatan sulfate on thrombin inhibition in human plasma. *J Clin Med* 117, 359, 1991.
41. **Naito, K., Fujikawa, K.** Activation of human blood coagulation Factor XI independent of Factor XII. *J Biol Chem* 266, 7353, 1991.
42. **Gailani, D., Broze, G.J., Jr.** Factor XII-independent activation of Factor XI in plasma: effects of sulfatides on tissue Factor-induced coagulation. *Blood* 82, 813, 1993.
43. **Broze, G.J., Jr.** The role of tissue Factor pathway inhibitor in a revised coagulation cascade. *Semin Hematol* 29, 159, 1992.
44. **Ofosu, F.A., Barrowcliffe, T.W.** Mechanisms of action of low molecular weight heparins and heparinoids. *Baillières Clin Haematol* 3, 505, 1990.
45. **Ofosu, F.A., Fenton, J.W., II, Maraganore, J., Blajchman, M.A., Yang, X., Smith, L.M., Anvari, N., Buchanan, M.R., Hirsh, J.** Inhibition of the amplification reactions of blood coagulation by

site specific inhibitors of thrombin. *Biochem J* 283, 893, 1992.
46. **Yang, X., Blajchman, M.A., Craven, S., Smith, L.M., Anvari, N., Ofosu, F.A.** Activation of Factor V during intrinsic and extrinsic coagulation. Inhibition by heparin, hirudion and H-D-Phe-Pro-ArgCH_2Cl. *Biochem J* 272, 399, 1990.
47. **Esmon, C.T.** Molecular events that control the protein C anticoagulant pathway. *Thromb Haemost* 70, 29, 1993.
48. **Esmon, C.T., Esmon, N.L., Harris, K.V.** Complex formation between thrombin and thrombomodulin inhibits both thrombin-catalyzed fibrin formation and Factor V activation. *J Biol Chem* 257, 7944, 1982.
49. **Stone, S.R., Hofsteenge, J.** Kinetics of the inhibition of thrombin by hirudin. *Biochem* 25, 4622, 1986.

Chapter 2

THE STRUCTURAL BASIS FOR THROMBIN INHIBITION BY HIRUDIN AND SERPINS

Milton T. Stubbs and Wolfram Bode

I. INTRODUCTION

The action of thrombin is central to the processes of thrombosis and hemostasis. Thrombin (EC 3.4.21.5) exhibits both enzymatic and hormone-like properties, that can be both pro- and anti-coagulant (Fig. 1). Through the cleavage of fibrinogen, thrombin is a primary promoter of coagulation; the resulting fibrin polymerizes to form a matrix for the nascent clot. Thrombin activates a number of other coagulation factors such as V, VIII, XI and XIII via limited proteolysis (see Ref.[1] for a review). Factor XIIIa, which covalently cross-links fibrin, is activated by thrombin. Platelet aggregation, for which thrombin is the most potent stimulator, is effected by the thrombin induced activation of the thrombin receptor.[2,3] In addition, thrombin performs a number of anticoagulatory functions. On binding to the cell surface protein thrombomodulin, thrombin is modified to activate protein C, which, in turn, is responsible for the inactivation of Factors Va and VIIIa.[4]

Thrombin's enzymatic activity is under the control of only a few endogenous inhibitors such as α_2-macroglobulin, the serpins antithrombin III[5] and heparin cofactor II[6], and protease nexin I.[7] Binding to serpins is enhanced considerably by the acidic glycosaminoglycan heparin.[8] Hirudin, the anticoagulant found in the saliva of the medicinal leech, binds even more tightly, inhibiting thrombin directly.[9-12] Recently, a number of peptide thrombin inhibitors have also been isolated including haemadin from the Indian leech[13], the Kazal-type inhibitor rhodniin from the Mexican leech[14], and bothrojaracin from a viper venom.[15]

A variety of cellular effects of thrombin have been observed that might mediate inflammatory and reparative responses to vascular injury: it induces platelet aggregation and stimulates secretion, acts as a mitogen for fibroblasts and macrophage-like cells and exhibits chemotactic properties.[16,17]

Recent studies have shown that thrombin is also involved in processes of brain development and maintenance. The interplay of thrombin, which causes neurite retraction in nerve cells, and protease nexins I and II, which reverse the process, point to an important

0-8493-7649-1/95/$0.00+$.50

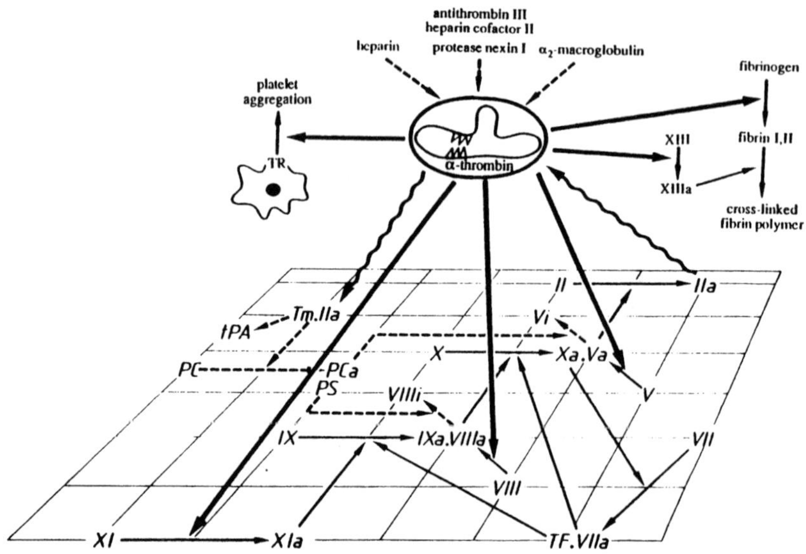

Figure 1. Thrombin and hemostasis. Release of thrombin (also termed Factor IIa) into the blood vessel is the result of the (predominantly membrane located calcium dependent) cascade reactions, which begin upon tissue damage with complex formation of Factor VII and tissue factor (TF). Blood factors are denoted by their roman numerals; activated factors carry the suffix "a". Bold arrows show thrombin proteolytic action. Cleavage of fibrinogen results in fibrin clot formation; that of the thrombin receptor (TR) leads to various cellular responses, including platelet aggregation. Anticoagulatory functions are denoted by dashed arrows. The thrombin inhibitory effects of the serpins are accelerated by heparin. Upon forming a complex with the surface-bound thrombomodulin (Tm), thrombin activates protein C (PC), which in conjunction with protein S (PS) inactivates members of the procoagulatory pathway (inactivated factors carry the suffix "i"). Cells exhibiting thrombin-bound thrombomodulin are stimulated to produce tissue plasminogen activator (tPA).

function in making and maintaining nerve cells connections. These neural functions are in addition to the normal coagulatory functions necessary for blood-brain barrier maintenance.[18]

The X-ray crystallographic structure of α-thrombin[19,20] has thrown light on this "multifunctional specificity". Considerable additional structural information is now available, including the structural requirements of thrombin when complexed with hirudin[21-24], fibrinopeptide A[26,27] or the prothrombin kringle fragment F2[28]; with inhibitors directed towards the active site[29-35], the exosite[25,36,37,40] or both[25,38-40]; and for prothrombin Gla and kringle F1 domain[41,42]

Table 1
Experimental X-ray crystallographic structures of thrombin.

Ligand	Resolution (Å)	Reference	
1. Thrombin — PPACK	1.9	Bode et al., 1989	19
		Bode et al., 1992	20
2. Thrombin — hirudin	2.3	Rydel et al., 1990	21
		Rydel et al., 1991	22
	2.9	Grütter et al., 1990	23
(bovine)	2.8	Vitali et al., 1992	24
3. Thrombin — peptides			
hirugen, hirulog1	2.2	Skrzypczak et al., 1991	25
fibrinopeptide A-hirudin (54-65)	2.5	Stubbs et al., 1992	26
fibrinopeptide A (bovine)	2.3	Martin et al., 1992	27
4. Thrombin — prothrombin F2	3.2	Arni et al., 1993	28
5. Thrombin — active site inhibitors			
(trypsin)	1.8	Bode et al., 1990	29
(trypsin)		Turk et al., 1991	30
(trypsin)	2.5	Matsuzaki et al., 1989	31
(bovine)	2.3	Brandstetter et al., 1992	32
	3.0	Banner and Hadvary, 1991	33
peptidomimetic inhibitor	2.5	Wu et al., 1993	34
cyclotheonamide A	2.3	Maryanoff et al., 1992	35
6. Thrombin — exosite inhibitors			
hirullin, MDL-28050	2.2	Qiu et al., 1993	36
DNA aptamer	2.9	Padmanabhan et al.,1993	37
7. Thrombin — bivalent inhibitors			
hirulog 3	2.3	Qiu et al., 1992	38
hirutonins 2 and 6	2.0	Zdanov et al., 1993	39
hirudin derivatives	2.2	Priestle et al., 1993	40
8. Prothrombin fragments			
apo F1 prothrombin fragment	2.25	Seshadri et al.,1991	41
CaF1 prothrombin fragment	2.5	Soriano-Garcia et al., 1992	42

(Table 1), Factor Xa[44] and serpins[94-103] (Table 2). Understanding these structural interactions has led to the understanding of the many interactions of thrombin at an atomic level.

In this chapter, we have focused on the experimental crystallographic structures of α-thrombin, and have related them to its multiple functions. In addition, we have highlighted the interactions with fibrinogen, hirudin, and the serpins antithrombin III and heparin cofactor II. For a more complete review of the relationship of thrombin structure to function, and its interactions with other proteins and small inhibitors, the reader is referred to Ref.[17]

Table 2
X-ray crystallographic structures of serpins.

Serpin	Resolution (Å)	Reference	
Cleaved α_1-proteinase inhibitor	3.0	Lobermann et al., 1984	94
Cleaved α_1PI, S-variant	3.1	Engh et al., 1989	95
Cleaved ovalbumin (plakalbumin)	2.8	Wright et al., 1990	96
Intact ovalbumin	2.0	Stein et al., 1990	97
Cleaved α_1-antichymotrypsi	3.0	Baumann et al.,1991	98
Cleaved leukocyte elastase inhibitor	2.0	Baumann et al.,1992	99
Latent plasminogen activator inhibitor	2.6	Mottonen et al.,1992	100
Cleaved antithrombin III	3.2	Mourey et al., 1993	101
Intact α_1-antichymotrypsin	2.5	Wei et al., 1994	102
Intact antithrombin III	3.2	Schreuder et al., 1994	103

II. THROMBIN STRUCTURE AND ITS SITES OF INTERACTION

The α-thrombin molecule is a trypsin-like serine proteinase, generated by autocatalytic and Factor Xa cleavage of the circulating plasma protein prothrombin.[45] Prothrombin is synthesized in the liver, where it is extensively post-translationally modified, including glycosylation at three sites, and its amino terminal domain is modified in a vitamin K-dependent manner to introduce γ-carboxyglutamate residues. Under physiological conditions, prothrombin associates with negative charged phospholipid surfaces in the presence of calcium. On the membrane, prothrombin combines with the prothrombinase complex comprising Factor Xa, Va and phospholipid, held together with calcium.[46] Factor Xa cleavage of prothrombin liberates the enzymatically active α-thrombin. The membrane surface activation localizes the production of thrombin to the site of injury.[47,48] Fragments of the prothrombin molecule have been determined crystallographically [28,41,42], as has the structure of Factor Xa[44], but these will not be dealt with here (see Refs.[17,49]).

The mature enzyme consists of two polypeptides, the 36 residue A- and 259 residue B-chains in human[50], covalently linked by a disulfide bridge. Like trypsin, thrombin cleaves after basic PI residues, with a clear preference for arginine and a narrower substrate specificity, however (Pn, Sn denote the nth substrate/proteinase site N-terminal to the cleavage site; similarly, Pn, Sn denote those sites C-terminal to the cleavage bond).[51] An apolar patch distant from the active site has been shown to contribute significantly to enzymatic activities[52], and a positive-charged region remote from the point of cleavage has been implicated in many thrombin-driven processes.[53]

A. OVERALL STRUCTURE

The globular α-thrombin molecule, depicted in Plate 1, is an ellipsoid of approximate dimensions 45 x 45 x 50 $Å^3$, with a deep canyon in which the active site is located.[19,20] Figure 2 (see page 24) provides a schematic representation of the major interaction sites of α-thrombin.[17] The approximate location of surface residues contributing to the various sites is shown. The active site cleft, with the catalytic residues at its base, runs from "west" to "east", where a substrate molecule would bind from amino to carboxy terminal. A prominent fork in the cleft is apparent immediately after the active site triad, resulting in a "northern" exit to the canyon.[19,26]

As with other members of the serine proteinase family, thrombin divides into two essentially six-stranded barrel domains held together by four transdomain straps, with five helical segments, one helical turn, and various surface located turn structures. The boomerang-shaped A-chain, with its multiple turns and short C-terminal helix, lies in a groove of the B-chain at the back of the molecule (opposite to the active site). The catalytic residues Ser195, His57 and Asp102 (chymotrypsinogen numbering)[17,19,20] are located at the junction between the two barrels. Characteristic of thrombin are several insertions with respect to trypsin (denoted by letter suffixes) which surround the active site cleft, making it deeper and narrower (Plate 1). The active site is therefore far less accessible to macromolecular substrates, a primary cause for the narrow specificity of α-thrombin.

The active site canyon is closed on the northern edge by the Tyr60A-Pro60B-Pro60C-Trp60D insertion loop (the "60 loop"). This sequence, unique to thrombin, is absolutely conserved in the 11 thrombin sequences known to date.[54] The loop is relatively rigid, deviating less than 1Å in the various structures determined. This small degree of movement is correlated with the binding of different molecules, as the loop forms an hydrophobic "lid" to the active site. Model building studies[19,20] suggest that most "small" protein inhibitors[43] would collide with this loop, explaining their generally observed weak affinity for thrombin. This loop restricts the approach of most possible protein substrates, giving the thrombin molecule extra discrimination for proteolytic action. Recent experiments with thrombin mutants lacking the Pro60B-Trp60D segment confirm this view.[55] The nine residue insertion between Leu60 and Glu61 also contains the point of carbohydrate attachment, Asn60G. Although the side chain of this residue is well defined in the PPACK-thrombin crystal, no interpretable electron density is observed for the carbohydrate chain, indicating that it extends away from the active site cleft in agreement with the lack of any effect on enzymatic and cellular activities of thrombin upon its removal.[17,20]

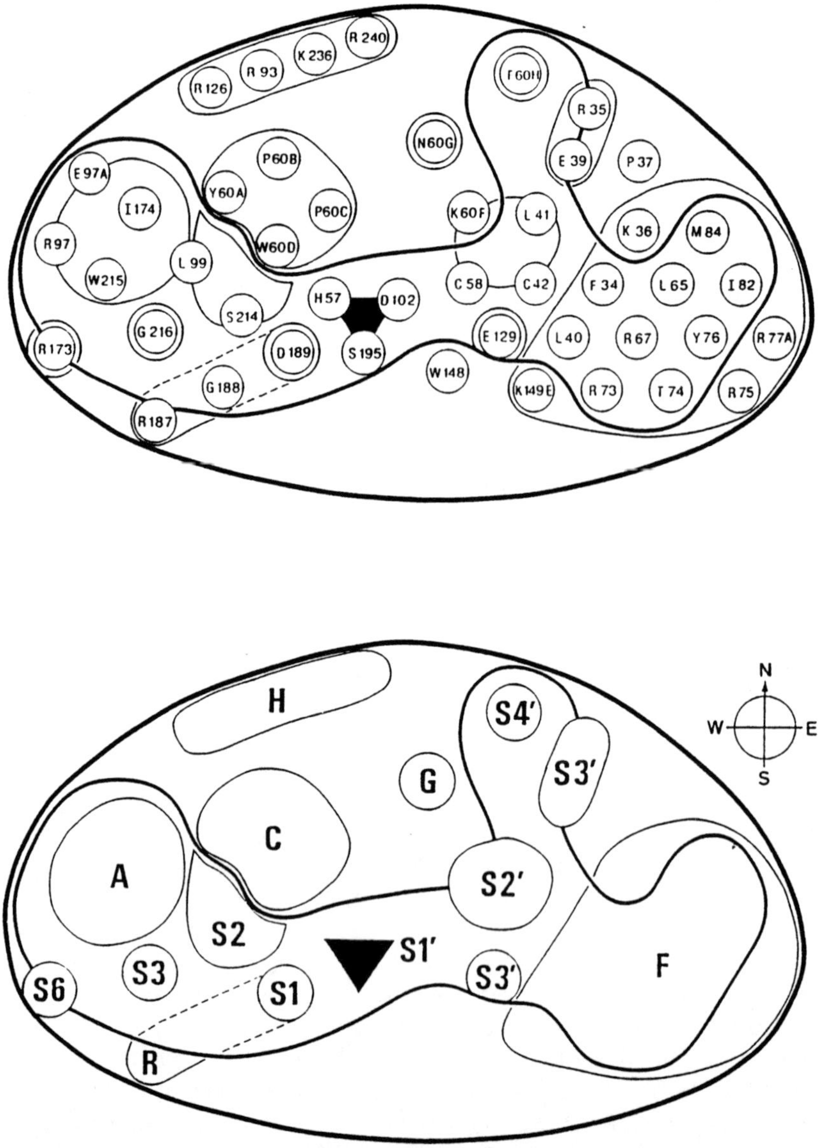

Figure 2. Schematic diagram showing residues involved in the various subsites of thrombin.[17] Surface residues appear in their approximate locations in the standard orientation (top) (see Plate 1). Lower part shows the division of the surface into functional regions. Key: ▾ — active site triad; S1 > S6 — specificity sites N-terminal to cleavage; A — aryl-binding site; F — fibrinogen recognition exosite; H — heparin binding site; G — glycosylation site; S1'->S3' — putative specificity sites C-terminal to cleavage; C — chemotactic region; R-RGD sequence; compass — defines orientation relative to active centre.

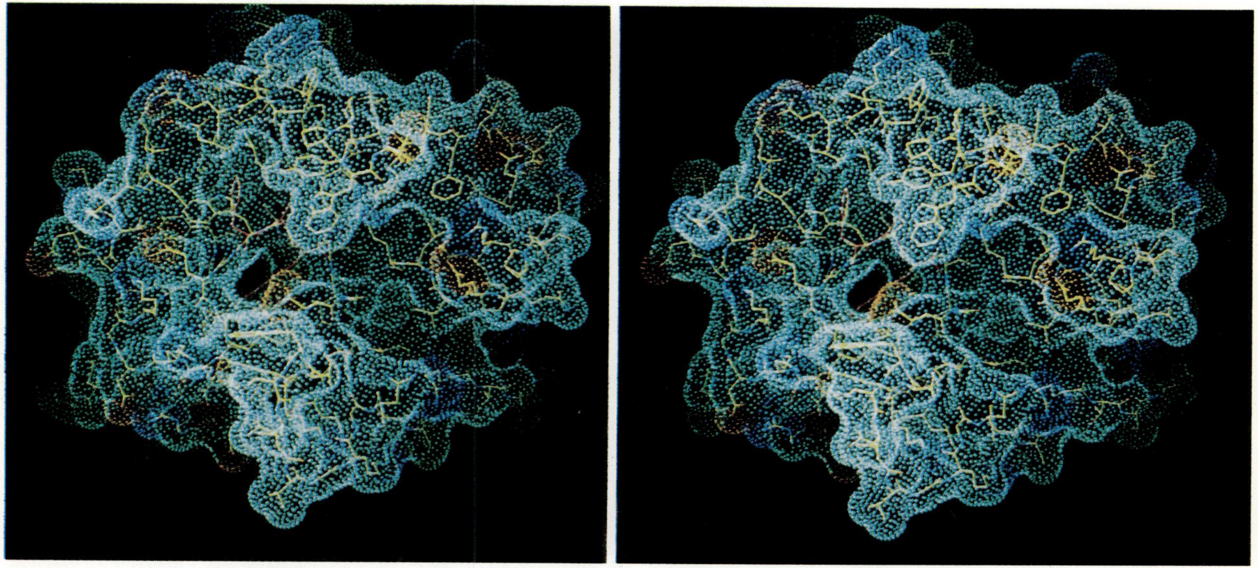

PLATE 1. Stereo view of the active site cleft of human α-thrombin,[20] displayed with a Connolly dot surface; molecular surfaces are coloured dark blue, red, and light blue if donated by basic, acidic or other residues, respectively. The bound PPACK molecule is show in red, with its Arg3' side chain disappearing into the "hole" in the surface close to the centre; this corresponds to the entrance to the specificity pocket. This view defines the "standard" orientation, with the active-site cleft of the B-chain running from left to right ("west-east", see Figure 2), the direction in which a substrate polypeptide chain would run. Only the front parts of the thrombin molecule and its molecular surface are displayed. The "60-insertion loop", in particular Trp60D, partially occludes the active site to the "north"; the "fibrinogen recognition exosite" is to the "east".

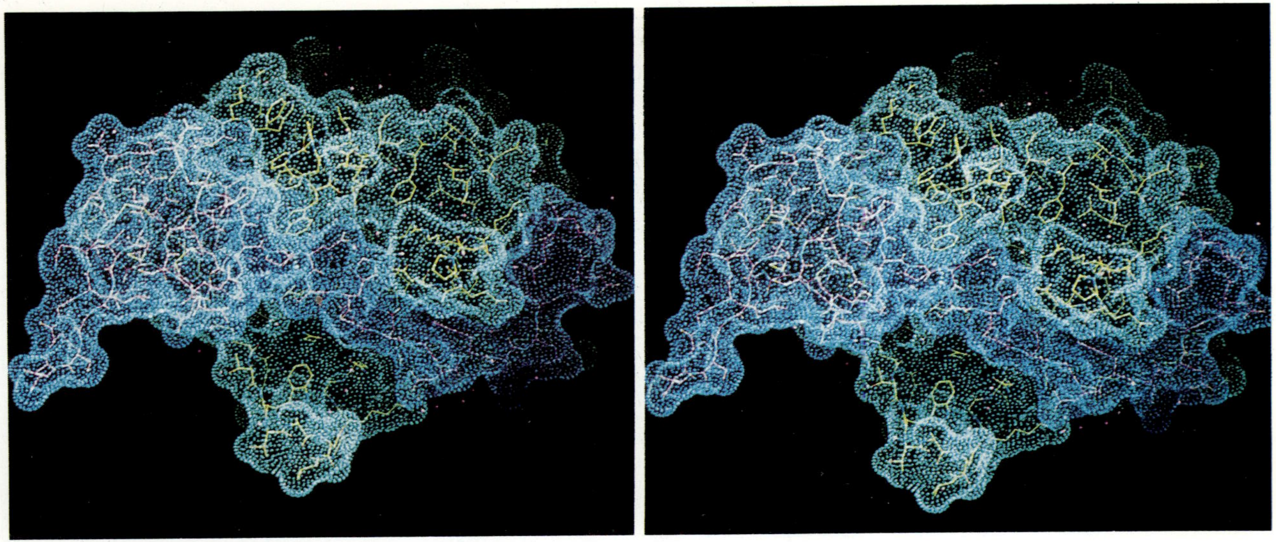

PLATE 2. The interaction between recombinant hirudin (red) and human α-thrombin (yellow) displayed together with their Connolly dot surfaces (blue and green, respectively) in the standard orientation.[17,22] The globular N-terminal disulphide knotted globular domain (stereo) of hirudin sits over the active site, rendering it inaccessible to macromolecular substrates. The C-terminal acidic tail stretches along the fibrinogen recognition exosite (see also Figure 4). This tail is flexible in the free hirudin molecule.

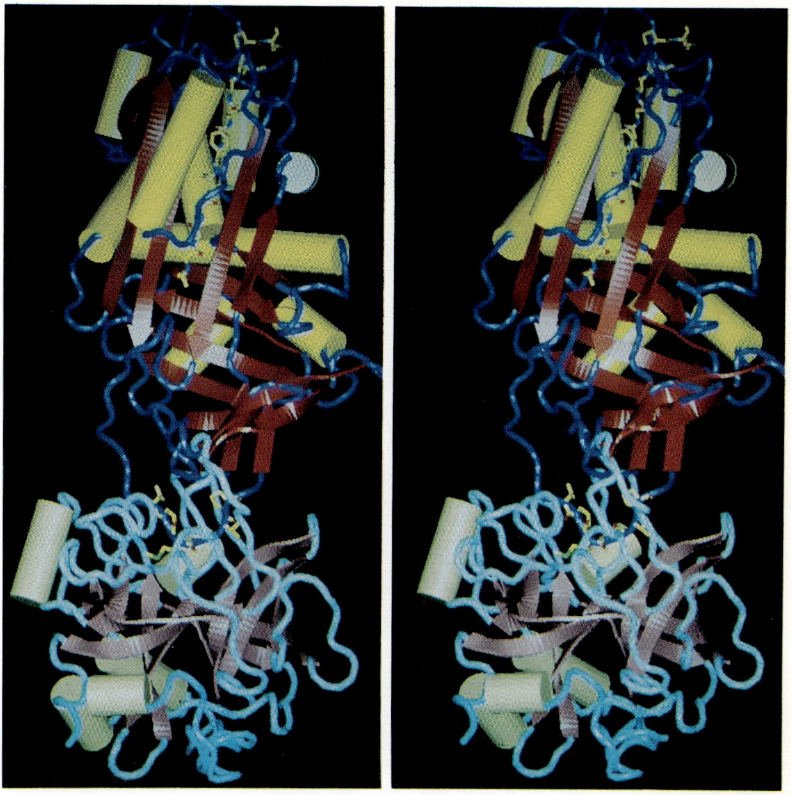

PLATE 3. Hypothetical complex of human α-thrombin (light colours) and an active serpin inhibitor (bold colours) in ribbon representation.[90] View is from the "south" (Plate 1 and Figure 2), such that the "148-insertion loop" is at the front, i.e., corresponding to the standard orientation by a rotation of 90° about a horizontal axis. The active site loop of the serpin (blue ribbon) runs from the left to right along thrombin's active site cleft. As no structure is available for a serpin with inhibitory activity, this complex has been modelled according to data for an active binary complex of α1-proteinase inhibitor and undecapeptide P1-P11 in sheet A front (in stick representation).[108] In cleaved serpins, the position of the peptide is occupied by residues of the new N-terminus formed on active site cleavage; in native serpins, the two β-strands shown on either side of the peptide presumably anneal together. The active site loop, modelled according to the canonical conformation of serine proteinase inhibitors, slots into the active site cleft of thrombin. The heparin binding site of antithrombin III and heparin cofactor II would be around the large helix A (back, horizontal) and helix D (to the left of and perpendicular to helix A at the back of the molecule). This is near to the heparin binding site of thrombin (back left). The fibrinogen recognition exosite, used by heparin cofactor II, is to the right. Figure courtesy of Dr. R.A. Engh.

On the south rim, a five-residue insertion near Trp148 opposes the YPPW loop. Although well defined in the PPACK-thrombin[20], the hirudin-thrombin structures[21-23], and hirudin derivative structures [25,26,40], it is found in differing conformations in each. Thus, in contrast to the "60 loop", this loop can exhibit multiple conformations and is able to move as a rigid body about Glu146 and Gly149E. Displacement of this loop or flap from its position in the PPACK-thrombin structure is required for the binding of hirudin. Deletion of residues Glu146-Trp148 dramatically alters thrombin interactions with serine proteinase inhibitors, and drastically reduces clotting activity[56], suggesting that this loop may play more than a merely passive role in thrombin interactions.

B. ELECTROSTATIC PROPERTIES

The tertiary arrangement of α-thrombin gives rise to a distinctive electrostatic potential.[20,57] In human thrombin, the A- and B-chains possess a large number of ionizable groups[89] at pH 7, ten of which are completely buried and inaccessible to bulk water. The isoelectric point of human α-thrombin is slightly above neutral, in agreement with an almost balanced number of acidic and basic residues. These are distributed non-uniformly, however, with positive charges concentrated in two "poles" to the east and northwest, between which the negative charges are sandwiched. The clustering of charged residues that are not properly balanced by neighbouring counter charges gives rise to a series of positive and negative charged surface patches. Presumably these are responsible for the unusual binding of thrombin to cation exchange resins and to negative charged surfaces. Some of the residues in these clusters have a destabilizing effect on the molecule, counteracted by residues peripheral to the clusters that are largely involved in salt bridges.

The distribution of charge in the thrombin molecule results in high positive and negative electrostatic field strengths outside the surface of the thrombin molecule.[57] Three specific surface patches, two positive and one negative charged, have received particular attention. One region of high positive charge density extends along the convex thrombin surface between Lys149E and Lys110 to the "east" of the active site, termed the "anion-binding exosite I" or "fibrinogen recognition exosite".[53] In this article, we shall use the latter designation. A large negative charged surface patch extends around the active site of thrombin. The two patches result in a bipolar charge distribution along the active site cleft, which would clearly influence the orientation of approaching substrates and inhibitors of large electric moments, such as hirudin. The strongest positive electrostatic field is observed for a groove on the "north" face of the thrombin molecule near its C-terminus. As this region interacts with heparin [58,59], it is termed the "heparin binding site", although it could alternatively be termed "anion binding exosite II" (see below and Ref.[20]).

The charged groups of thrombin are therefore not simply for structural stabilization; those that do not contribute to the overall stability perform other essential functions. The unfavourable electrostatic interactions observed are tolerated in order to create strong external electrostatic fields for interactions with external ligands; they represent an "energy reserve", to be used by the protein to select and bind substrates and inhibitors.

C. ACTIVE SITE GEOMETRY, PRE-CLEAVAGE SITES (S1-S3, ARYL-BINDING SITE), AND PRIMED SITES (S1'-S3')

The active site triad Ser195-His57-Asp102 of thrombin displays a geometry virtually indistinguishable from that of the other members of the trypsin-like serine proteinase family. The free amino terminus of Ile16, formed only on proteolytic cleavage of the A- and B-chains, makes an internal salt bridge with Asp194, thereby playing a crucial role in the formation of the active site. Comparison of the active site of PPACK-thrombin,[20] where Arg3' is covalently attached to Ser195 and His57 with the free active site of hirugen-thrombin[25], shows that the geometry of Ser195 is only slightly affected by the tetrahedral hemiketal arrangement (nomenclature: in this chapter, substrate/ inhibitor residue numbers bear an apostrophe as suffix, e.g. Arg3' of PPACK, unless otherwise stated).

The S1-S3 sites in PPACK-thrombin are occupied in an antiparallel fashion by Arg3', Pro2', and D-Phe1', respectively (Fig. 3). The primary specificity site S1 is practically identical to that of trypsin, with Asp189 at the bottom of the pocket positioned to make a salt bridge with basic P1 residues. The only difference seen in the S1 pocket is the substitution of trypsin Ser190 for thrombin Ala190. The S1 pocket of thrombin is therefore slightly less polar, with one less hydrogen bond accepter/donor. The larger space and lack of a hydrogen bond partner suggest that a lysyl side chain would not bind as tightly, explaining the differential affinities of thrombin for arginine and lysine P1 residues.[20]

The pyrrolidine ring of Pro2' of PPACK sits in a hydrophobic pocket formed by residues His57, Ser214, Leu99, Tyr60A, and Trp60D, with the latter two residues forming a lid to the pocket. This S2 site is ideally suited to the binding of medium sized non-polar residues, explaining their frequent occurrence as P2 residues in thrombin macromolecular substrates (Table 3, see page 28), and the particular reactivity of chloromethylketone inhibitors with P2 proline residues.[60]

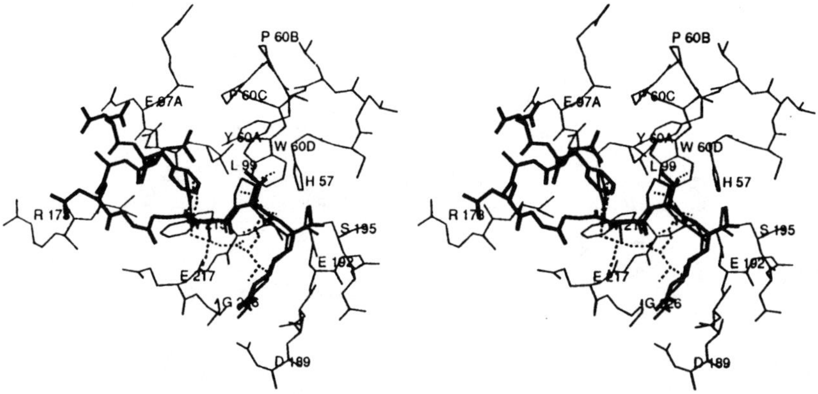

Figure 3. Interactions of fibrinopeptide A[26] (bold), DPhe-Pro-Arg-MeCl[20] (medium) and hirudin[22] (dashed) in the active site of thrombin in standard orientation (stereo). Arg3' of **PPACK** forms a tetrahedral hemiketal structure covalently linked to Ser195 Oγ and His57 Nδ, with simultaneous salt bridge formation with Asp189 (S1); Pro2' binds tightly into the S2 cavity; DPhe1' makes two antiparallel main chain hydrogen bonds to Gly216 (S3 interaction), and, due to its D-configuration, its benzyl ring nestles into the hydrophobic "aryl-binding site" simultaneously. Phe8' and Leu9' of **fibrinopeptide A** occupy the aryl-binding site, approaching Vall5' in the S2 site, filling the hydrophobic apolar binding site; the benzyl ring of Phe8' occupies the aryl-binding site similarly to DPhe1' of PPACK, but from the opposite direction due to the intricate folding. The specificity pocket is unoccupied by **hirudin**, although the side chain of Thr2' points towards it; the N-terminal hirudin segment Ile1'-Tyr3' runs parallel to thrombin segment Ser214-Gly219; Ile1' occupies the S2 subsite, with its amino group in hydrogen bond distance to His57 Nε and Ser195 Oγ; and Tyr3' occupies the aryl-binding site.

The S2 site abuts a second hydrophobic pocket, lined by residues Ile174, Trp215,and segment 97-99. Occupied by the D-Phe1' benzyl ring of PPACK, this region is particularly suited to aromatic residues. Presumably, the perpendicular aryl-aryl (edge-on) arrangement and aryl-carbonyl contact with the carbonyl group of Glu97A seen for D-Phe1' of PPACK[20], Tyr3' of hirudin[21], Phe8' of fibrinopeptide A[26], and the aromatic moieties of various small inhibitors[32,33] contribute considerably to the binding strength of these peptides. This site therefore, is termed the aryl-binding site[29], to distinguish it from the S2 cavity. These two sites have alternatively been termed D (distal) and P (proximal) sites,respectively.[33] The two comprise a single common hydrophobic surface, forming the apolar binding site identified previously.[52] The residues contributing to the apolar binding site named above are nearly all absolutely conserved between species.[54] Those that are not, show conservative substitutions, pointing to the

Table 3. Cleavage sites of thrombin substrates and downstream acidic sequences that (could) bind to the fibrinogen recognition exosite. "n" denotes the number of residues between P4' and the start of the sequence shown. P1 residual underlined; negatively charged residues hold; hydrophobic groups italic. Y* indicates sulphated Tyr.

Substrate	P4	P3	P2	P1	P1'	P2'	P3'	P4'	"n"	Acidic Sequence
Fibrinogen Aα	7DFLAGG	G	V	R	G	P	R	V	13	W F C S D E D W N Y K C P S G C
Fibrinogen Bβ	11F	S	A	R	G	H	R	P	46	C L H A D P D L G V L C P T G C
Fibrinogen γ										8C C I L D E R F G S Y C P T T C
Factor V	706L	G	I	R	S	F	R	N	5	L N Q E E E E F
Factor V	1015L	S	P	R	T	F	H	P		
Factor V	1542W	Y	L	R	S	N	N	G	24	D I E D S D D I P E D
Factor VIII	369I	Q	I	R	S	V	A	K	11	A E E E D W D Y A P L
Factor VIII	737I	E	P	R	S	F	S	Q	16	I P E N D I E K T D P
Factor VIII	1686Q	S	P	R	S	F	Q	K		
Factor XI	366I	K	P	R	I	V	G	G		
Factor XIII	35V	V	P	R	G	V	N	L		
Thrombin receptor	38L	D	P	R	S	F	L	L	4	D K Y E P F W E D E E K N E S G
Protein C	166V	D	P	R	L	I	D	G		
Thrombomodulin										408E C P E G Y I L D D G F I C T D I D E
Antithrombin III	390I	A	G	R	S	L	N	P		
Heparin cofactor II	441F	M	P	L	S	S	T	Q	(-395)	53E G E E D D D Y* L D L E K I F S E D D D Y* I D
Protease nexin I	342L	I	A	R	S	S	P	P		
Hirudin										54G D F E E I P E E Y* L Q

importance of this region in the action of thrombin.

D-Phe1' of PPACK makes a two-rung ß-ladder with Gly216. This P3-S3 interaction is similar to that observed in the "canonical" serine proteinase-inhibitor interaction[43], i.e. antiparallel ß-sheet formation between a loop of the inhibitor and the enzyme. That the P3 residue of PPACK is of D-configuration indicates that it can insert its aromatic benzyl ring directly into the aryl-binding site simultaneously. This is not the case for normal substrates or inhibitors, where an L-configured P3-residue would extend away from the active site to interact with another thrombin site. Instead, the P4 side chain of a bound all L-amino acid polypeptide substrate would point towards this hydrophobic cleft (Table 3). Such an interaction has recently been inferred from NMR experiments on thrombin receptor peptides with thrombin.[61] This suggests that the P4 Leu residue occupies this position. The beneficial effect of large bulky aromatic residues at P4 connected to a P3-glycine has been used to construct suitable thrombin substrates.[62]

Due to little direct structural evidence, the primed subsites (C-terminal to cleavage) of thrombin cannot be described with a confidence equivalent to the unprimed sites, and are probably not unique (see Ref.[17]). The S1' subsite of thrombin is limited in size due to the impeding Lys60F, and therefore is particularly suited for small P1' residues such as glycine or alanine (or even serine or aspartate). This is consistent with the frequent occurrence of small P1' residues in natural protein substrates. The primed sites have been modelled for fibrinogen[26], which allows a model for the thrombomodulin-mediated cleavage of protein C (Fig. 4, see next page). Slightly different sites are observed for these residues in the non-cleavable hirulog 3 and hirutonin 6.[38,39]

D. THE FIBRINOGEN RECOGNITION EXOSITE

The positive charged patch to the "east" has been identified as the fibrinogen recognition exosite (Figs. 2 and 4). The field is centred around thrombin loop Lys70-Glu80 (the structure of which is stabilised by a number of salt bridges buried in an architecture similar to the "calcium binding loop" of trypsin), surrounded in space by several (sequentially distant) Lys and Arg residues. At the surface, residues Arg73, Arg75 and Arg77A of this loop are surrounded by Arg35, Lys36 and Lys149E; just below, Lys81, Lys109 and Lys110 contribute to the field. The positive charge is compensated for only partially by acidic residues Glu77 and Glu80, involved in a buried ionic cluster.

The exosite is involved in fibrinogen and thrombin receptor cleavage, in fibrin and thrombomodulin binding, in inhibition by hirudin, and in glycosaminoglycan-mediated heparin cofactor II binding (see

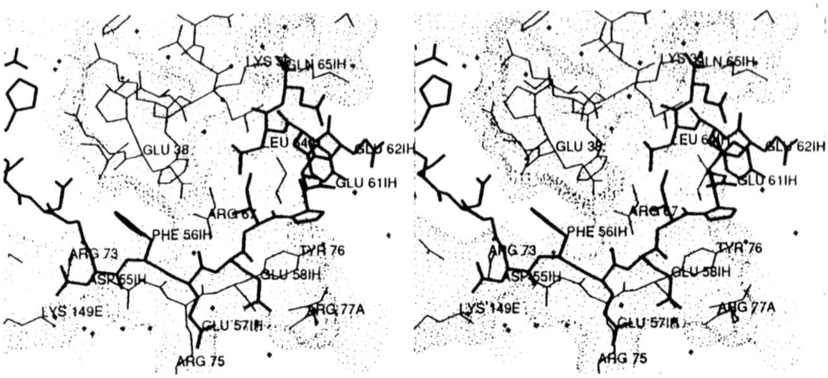

Figure 4. The fibrinogen recognition exosite of thrombin (thin connections) and the carboxy-terminal hirudin segment (thick connections) of thrombin-hirudin[22], displayed together with the Connolly surface of thrombin, in standard orientation (stereo). The tail of hirudin is in an extended conformation, ending with a 3_{10}-helix, and fits snugly into the fibrinogen recognition exosite. The large number of acidic residues of hirudin and of basic residues of thrombin can be seen. At the right is Tyr63', which is sulphated in wild-type hirudins.

Refs.[17,20]). Common to these peptide sequences is a string of negatively charged residues with little or no conventional sequence homology (Table 3). The crystal structures of hirudin in its complex with α-thrombin[21-24] reveals that the carboxy terminal acidic tail occupies the fibrinogen recognition exosite. The conformation of this carboxy terminal peptide is independent of the rest of the hirudin molecule.[25,26] These have provided insights into the salient features of interactions at this site (Fig. 4).

The hirudin tail binds in an extended conformation, ending with a short 3_{10}-helix. The interaction is of a dual nature: part ionic, between acidic residues of hirudin and basic residues of thrombin, flanked by (two semi-contiguous) hydrophobic patches. Considering the large number of charged residues, remarkably few direct hydrogen bond/salt bridges are made in this region; in particular the two acidic hirudin residues Glu61' and Glu62' do not contact the enzyme. Rather than utilizing one-to-one inter-residual contacts, binding is stabilized by a more general complementarity of electrostatic fields. This is borne out by the close agreement between electrostatic model calculations and mutant hirudin inhibition studies.[63-65] The field complementarity negates the need for employing specific salt bridge interactions. This would suggest an "exosite consensus" sequence of several negative charged residues interspersed with bulky hydrophobic residues, the latter anchoring the charged peptides in the apolar crevices that line the fibrinogen recognition exosite.

E. THE HEPARIN BINDING SITE

The other positive charged region has been assigned as the heparin binding site, in agreement with chemical modification data[58,66] and recent mutagenesis data.[59] Centred around the side chains of Arg93, Arg126, Lys236 and Lys240 on the "northern" edge of the molecule (Fig. 3), this patch extends over the surface as far as the "west" face, encompassing the basic residues Arg97, Arg101, Arg165, Lys169, Arg172, Arg175, Arg233 and Lys235. The observed high affinity binding of heparin to thrombin[67] might be accomplished through the favourable electrostatic interactions between this patch and the linear large negative field of the former, coupled with specific recognition sites.

Heparin (and other sulphated glycosaminoglycans) are important regulators of blood coagulation (reviewed in Ref.[68]). Heparin accelerates complex formation of thrombin with the serpins antithrombin III[5] and heparin cofactor II[6] (see below). Inactivation of thrombin by antithrombin III is impaired by the binding of the latter to prothrombin fragment F2[69], which binds to the heparin binding site.[28] This confers the advantage that thrombin is not inhibited in the early stages of coagulation. The heparin binding site also plays a role in the interaction with thrombomodulin, the chondroitin sulphate moiety of which provides a secondary low affinity site for thrombin.[70] There is some evidence that, in the absence of antithrombin III, heparin will bind to both the fibrinogen recognition exosite and to the heparin binding site.[71] Similarly, fibrin may interact with both sites, leading to sequestration of thrombin in the developing blood clot. Binding of fibrin at the heparin site would presumably leave the enzyme active. However, the major antithrombotic effect of heparin is attributable to suppression of the thrombin dependent amplification reactions, i.e. activation of Factors V and VIII.[72]

F. THE CHEMOTACTIC DOMAIN AND THE RGD REGION

Several thrombin-derived peptides have been implicated as mediators of cellular events (see Refs.[16,17]). The compact and rather rigid Tyr60A-Pro60B-Pro60C-Trp60D loop involved in extracellular matrix binding and chemotactic/growth factor activities may represent the chemotactic domain of thrombin. The RGD triplet Arg187-Gly188-Asp189 might play a part in platelet binding, for example, as a docking site for the extracellular matrix, facilitating thymidine incorporation by fibroblasts, and affecting mitogenesis and cell adhesion. Arg187 is the only side chain of this triplet on the surface of the molecule, and is involved in rather strong surface salt/hydrogen bond bridges; Gly188 is buried and Asp189 is at the bottom of the S1 site. To recognize the motif, presumably an approaching cellular receptor requires a partially unfolded thrombin molecule. Partial proteolytic degradation or thermal denaturation may play a part in this process. Alternatively, a zymogen-like (pro)thrombin species may be involved, where this peptide fragment could be turned "inside-out" as in chymotrypsinogen.[20] Parts of the heparin binding site (in particular, Lys169 and/or Lys240) might simultaneously act as a high affinity binding site for platelets.[66]

III. INTERACTION WITH FIBRINOGEN

Thrombin is able to cleave a number of small peptides, but shows a high degree of specificity when it comes to macromolecular substrates. Here we describe possible interactions of thrombin with fibrinogen, its major substrate.

Fibrinogen may be viewed as the prime target of thrombin enzymatic action. The 340 kDa molecule is a dimer of trimers with stoichiometry $(A\alpha,B\beta,\gamma)_2$. Thrombin cleavage results in the removal of the N-terminal fibrinopeptides A and B (16 and 14 residues in human, respectively, Table 2) to form fibrin, $(\alpha,\beta,\gamma)_2$. Unlike trypsin, thrombin has a very high specificity for this reaction; only four of the 376 Arg/Lys-Xaa bonds are cleaved in the native state. The Aα chain is the first and fastest to be cleaved; the first 51 residues of this chain are sufficient to mimic the fibrinopeptide A cleavage kinetics of fibrinogen.[73,74] Both the apolar binding site and the fibrinogen recognition exosite have been implicated in the exceptional specificity of this reaction (reviewed in Ref.[75]).

The ternary complex of human α-thrombin with peptides derived from fibrinopeptide A and hirudin[26] has allowed a structural explanation for this specificity. The decapeptide Asp7'-Arg16' exhibits a compact conformation (Fig. 3). The preceding six residues, not present in the crystal studied, would extend freely into solution. By making a hydrogen bond from the side chain carboxylate group of Asp7' to the backbone amide nitrogen of Ala10', a short stretch of irregularly hydrogen bonded α-helix is formed. The chain reverses its direction at Ala10', stabilised by intrapeptide main chain hydrogen bonds. The left-handed helical conformation of Gly12' is energetically unfavourable for non-glycyl residues. The remaining three residues Gly13'-Arg16' exhibit an extended β-strand conformation, with no intrapeptide hydrogen bonding. A similar fold was inferred previously from NMR measurements[76], but the proposed structure was overly compact; subsequent NMR measurements[26] confirmed the crystal structure.

The peptide structure is amphiphilic in nature, with a clustering of hydrophobic residues Phe8', Leu9' and Val15' to form a single surface, which slot into the apolar binding site of thrombin. Val15' occupies the S2 site, whilst Phe8' and Leu9' are in the aryl-binding site. Due to the opposite approach of the peptide chain, these two residues are able to fill the aryl-binding site much more fully than either Tyr3' of hirudin or D-Phe1' of PPACK. Analysis of mutated Aα1-50 fragment fusion proteins indicates that residues 7' to 16' of Aα are critical for efficient peptide hydrolysis, but are (surprisingly) less important to thrombin binding.[77] Hydrophobic contacts provide the majority of interactions, with only three intermolecular hydrogen bonds. The typical P3-S3 β-ladder described above for PPACK D-Phe1' also is seen between Gly14' and Gly216. Glu11' at P6 makes ionic contacts with Arg173 through the charged side groups. The small number of polar interactions observed in the fibrinopeptide A-thrombin structure presumably serve to anchor and/or orient the peptide correctly in the hydrophobic environment.

The thrombin cleavage of fibrinogen requires more than just fibrinopeptide recognition; the intact fibrinogen recognition exosite is also required. Hirudin, hirugen and hirudin (45'-65') are competitive inhibitors of fibrinogen cleavage.[78,79] As discussed above, the crystal structures of these complexes with thrombin suggest an "exosite consensus" of several negative charged residues, interspersed with bulky hydrophobic residues. The cleavage kinetics of fibrinopeptide A are almost completely accounted for by the first 51 residues of the fibrinogen Aα chain.[73,74] Residues 35'-43', with the sequence Phe-Cys*-Ser-Asp-Glu-Asp-Trp-Asn-Tyr, would appear to contain all the necessary features. A peptide containing residues 35'-43' inhibits fibrinogen cleavage competitively.[80] The Cys* residue is disulphide linked to Bβ Cys 65, and therefore must point away from the thrombin molecule.

This sequence is followed immediately by a conserved Cys-Xaa-Xaa-Xaa-Cys sequence, repeated in all three fibrinogen chains, which link the individual chains via disulphide bridges (Table 3). Analogous hydrophobic/acidic regions immediately precede the Cys-Xaa-Xaa-Xaa-Cys sequence in the Bβ and γ chains also, which could further enhance favourable electrostatic binding interactions (Fig. 5, see next page). The combined charge of the three chains may be important. The internal repetition of this sequence could imply a secondary (non-enzymatic) binding site for thrombin, although this second sequence is considerably less acidic.

There remain 18 residues between the Arg16' P1 residue and the

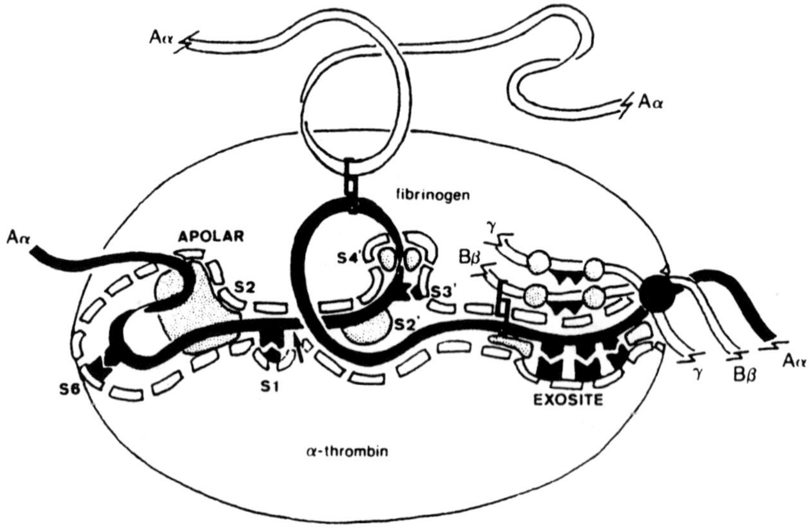

Figure 5. Schematic diagram showing the major interactions of the fibrinogen Aα chain (thick filled line) with thrombin.[26] The boundary of the active site cleft is depicted by a dashed line. Hydrophobic interactions are dotted, acidic groups depicted by ▲ and basic by . The cleavage point is marked by an arrow. Disulphide bridges connecting the individual fibrinogen chains are indicated by §; the Bβ and γ chains, linked by a disulphide knot (•), are shown in the neighbourhood of the fibrinogen recognition exosite.

putative exosite region of fibrinogen (Table 3). Residues P1' to P3' of fibrinogen Aα, Gly17'-Pro18'-Arg19', play a role in the cleavage process. Inspection of the putative S' sites allows modelling of these residues after the cleavage site with a reasonable conformation.[26] Gly17' (P1') is not required to make any special contacts. A depression in the surface of thrombin could accommodate the pyrrolidine ring of Pro18' (P2'). The Nζ group of Lys60F would be well placed to hydrogen bond with the carbonyl group of Pro18'. This site would appear to be well suited to small polar residues. This choice of S2' means that the substrate chain at P1'-P2' forks away from the main active site cleft occupied by hirudin (54'-65'). The chain therefore follows a course fundamentally different to that observed for canonical small serine proteinase inhibitors[43], which might explain the failure of docking experiments with such inhibitors.[19,20] This hypothetical choice of primed sites has been confirmed in essence in studies on the hirulog 3-thrombin complex.[38] The guanidinium group of Arg19' (P3') could be compensated for by a salt bridge to either Glu39 or Glu192, although the close approach of Arg35 to the former could interfere with such an interaction. After Arg19', the chain must exit the active site cleft. It is most likely that the substrate chain leaves through a depression in the active site wall formed between the characteristic thrombin surface loops containing residues Trp60D and Pro37A; to follow any other direction would partially occlude re-entry to the fibrinogen exosite. This would allow the favourable burial of Phe60H by the side chain of Val20' (P4'). The remaining (mainly polar) residues would then loop back across the active site cleft before entering the exosite.

After the first fibrinopeptide A has been cleaved off, thrombin could remain associated with the fibrin molecule via interactions at the fibrinogen recognition exosite. Cleavage of the second fibrinopeptide A and the two fibrinopeptides B could then be facilitated via limited diffusion. The colocalization of fibrin bound thrombin and Factor XIII[81] could also accelerate activation of the latter, initiating the cross-linking process. Sequestration of thrombin in the clot protects it from inactivation by serpins, increasing its active lifetime. Further protection may be afforded by additional fibrin binding to the heparin binding site.

IV. INTERACTION WITH HIRUDIN

Thrombin binds tightly to and is selectively inhibited by hirudin[9-11], a protein from the saliva of the medicinal leech *Hirudo medicinalis*. The major form of natural hirudin is a polypeptide of 65 amino acids, sulphated at Tyr63', with three disulphide bonds.[82] Hirudin reacts rapidly with thrombin to form a tight equimolar complex ($K_d = 10^{-14}$ M) (Ref.[10]). Recombinant forms not sulphated at Tyr63' exhibit a ten-fold reduced affinity for thrombin.[11] The structure of hirudin has been determined both in solution[83,84] and in crystal complexes with α-thrombin.[21-24] In solution, the N-terminal disulphide knotted domain forms a compact structure from Tyr3' to Lys47'; however, the first two residues, residues Gly31'-Gly36' and the carboxy terminal acidic tail, including in the wild type sulphated Tyr63', are disordered. In its complex with thrombin (Plate 2), the carboxy terminal three residues and the amino terminal tail become ordered, forming significant interactions with the enzyme.

The globular amino terminal domain consists of a four stranded β-structure centred on a three disulphide hydrophobic core. In complex with thrombin[22], the carboxy terminal tail of hirudin (48'-65') (disordered in the free molecule)[83,84] extends along the active site cleft to occupy the fibrinogen recognition exosite of thrombin, with a bend at Asp55' (Fig. 4 and Plate 2). The first part (Pro46'-His51') is organized in a polyproline II helix, ending with three residues of poorly defined density. From Asp55' to Pro60', the chain is an extended conformation, ending with Glu61' to Leu64' in a 3_{10} reverse turn. The disulphide domain sits over the active site, with the amino terminal situated in thrombin's active site. However, in contrast to substrate-like binding, the amino terminal residues Ile1'-Tyr3' form a *parallel* β-pleated structure with thrombin segment Ser214-Gly219 (Fig. 3). The catalytic Ser195 residue is hydrogen bonded to the free amino terminus of Ile1', which also forms a hydrogen bond to Ser214. The side chain of Ile1' occupies the hydrophobic S2 site, and the phenol ring of Tyr3' lies in the aryl-binding site. Thr2', at the entrance to the S1 specificity pocket, is too small to enter it to any significant amount, and cannot interact with Asp189. Instead, this pocket is occupied by ordered solvent molecules.[22] The interaction is enhanced by hirudin mutations of Thr2'->Arg[85], which allows salt bridge formation, and by Tyr3'->Phe or Trp, which allows more favourable interactions in the aryl-binding site.[86]

As described above, the acidic tail interacts with thrombin through numerous contacts, making up more than 1/3 of all hirudin-thrombin intermolecular contacts. Site-directed mutagenesis studies indicate that each of the five charged residues of recombinant hirudin contributes to complex stabilization.[65] This is in good agreement with electrostatic calculations, showing asymmetric and complementary electrostatic potentials around thrombin and hirudin.[63] The integrity of the fibrinogen recognition exosite is required for hirudin complexation, although catalytically active forms are not necessary. The hydrophobic interactions are certainly of importance, although the replacement of Phe56'->Ala, which makes an impressive number of intermolecular contacts, results in only slight effects on the binding constant.[65] In the hirugen-thrombin crystal structure[25], the sulphated Tyr63' residue occupies the same position as the unsulphated Tyr63' of recombinant hirudin-thrombin.[22] Surprisingly, the sulphate oxygen atoms make no ion pairs with opposite charged residues of thrombin; contacts are via direct and solvent mediated hydrogen bonds.

By sitting over the active site without directly contacting it (fundamentally different to "canonical" inhibition)[43], hirudin is able to hinder the approach of substrates to the active site. On approach of hirudin to thrombin in solution, the molecules may pre-orient themselves through the strong complementary electrostatic fields of the binding surfaces[63], accounting for the almost diffusion-controlled association rate constant.[11] The ionic strength dependence of kinetic parameters points to an initial association and rigidification of the negative charged tail of hirudin with the positive charged fibrinogen recognition exosite of thrombin. The amino-terminal domain would then bind over thrombin's active site via a favourable induced fit.

V. INTERACTION WITH SERPINS

In comparison to other serine proteinases, thrombin has very few endogenous conjugate protein inhibitors. In addition to the multifunctional α_2-macroglobulin, thrombin is inhibited by the serpins (serine proteinase inhibitors) antithrombin III,[19] heparin cofactor II[20] and proteinase nexin I.[21,22] α_1-Proteinase inhibitor (α_1PI), which serves as a paradigm for serpins with inhibitory activity, is primarily active against elastase; in the Pittsburg variant, however, a substitution of the PI Met358 for Arg renders potent antithrombin activity, resulting in a fatal bleeding disorder.[88]

Recent structural studies of the serpins have added much to our knowledge of their action (reviewed in Refs.[89,90]). According to thermodynamic and CD measurements[91-93], the active serpins exhibit two structurally distinct states. The uncleaved virgin inhibitors are thermodynamically less stable and display less secondary structure than their cleaved counterparts. Ovalbumin, a serpin with no inhibitory action, does not show this transition when it is cleaved to form plakalbumin.

Some serpins show so-called latency, where they are intact but inactive. X-ray crystallographic structures are now available for cleaved, intact and latent serpins (Table 2).[94-103]

Cleaved α_1PI consists of several helices and three large ß-sheets: a flat, six-stranded sheet A, a highly twisted six-stranded sheet B, and a twisted four-stranded sheet C (Plate 3).[94,85] The unprimed residues (those N-terminal to the cleavage) make up strand s4A of sheet A, whereas the primed residues align to sheet C. Surprisingly, the PI (Met358) and PI' (Ser359) residues are some 70Å apart in the cleaved α_1PI molecule (top and bottom of the molecule in Fig. 8, respectively). Clearly, substantial rearrangements must take place in secondary and tertiary structure on cleavage of α_1PI.

Some clarification of this has come through the structure determinations of plakalbumin[96] and ovalbumin.[97] Although the general structure of these molecules is similar to that of α_1PI, one important difference is seen. The large sheet A is one strand less with respect to α_1PI. In plakalbumin, strand s4A does not insert; in ovalbumin, it is linked to s1C with the central part organized as an helix. The lack of insertion appears to be primarily a result of the bulky side-chain Arg345 in ovalbumin/plakalbumin; in the active serpins, this residue is always small/hydrophobic.[89] Mutations of P14, P12 and P1 residues in α_1PI-like serpins result in inactive species.[104,105] This is also the case on insertion of a tetradecapeptide into α_1PI corresponding to residues P1-P14.[106] In the case of antithrombin III, insertion of the equivalent peptide results in an additional reduction in affinity for heparin.[107] That the insertion of a dodecameric peptide yields an active inhibitor suggests a role for the P14 residue.[108]

The inhibitory species of serpins, therefore, appear to have a character midway between the cleaved α_1PI form and the ovalbumin/plakalbumin structure. Evidence is accumulating that strand s4A is indeed partially inserted; the insertion of Thr345 appears sufficient to form the active form of α_1PI. The recently reported structure of intact antithrombin III suggests just such a structure[103], although intact α_1-antichymotrypsin shows no insertion[102], with an α-helical conformation of the active site loop as seen in ovalbumin.[97] In latent plasminogen activator inhibitor, strand s4A is fully inserted, with the primed sites now no longer part of sheet C.[100]

Mobility and differential insertion of the active site loop is a notable feature of serpin structure. Several lines of evidence indicate that the serpins bind to their cognate enzymes through an exposed binding loop of canonical conformation similar to that of the "small" serine proteinase inhibitors.[43] Furthermore, the interaction of this loop with thrombin is furthermore restricted to the immediate environment of the active site residues.[109-113] This loop has been modelled according to the canonical conformation, and docked with thrombin (Plate 3).[90]

Complex formation of thrombin with antithrombin III is accelerated by heparin[8], which might be accounted for by a "template mechanism".[68,114-116] If one assumes that the docking geometry above is correct, then the thrombin heparin binding site would be close to the presumed location of that in antithrombin III, i.e. helices A and D (Plate 3).[89] It is conceivable therefore that the tetradecameric heparin strand required links the two components, tightening the interaction.

The conditions for heparin cofactor II appear to be slightly different.[6,68] In contrast to other thrombin inhibitors, the P1 residue is Leu rather than Arg. In order to force this hydrophobic residue into the S1 pocket of thrombin, the inhibitor must bind more tightly elsewhere. In addition to a heparin binding site similar to antithrombin III, heparin cofactor II possesses a highly acidic N-terminal part (Table 3) which also plays a role in heparin (or dermatan sulphate) dependent complex formation.[109-113]

This N-terminus interacts with the fibrinogen recognition exosite[109,110], and is essential for heparin-mediated stimulation of thrombin inhibition.[109,112,113] It would seem that this acidic tail occupies heparin cofactor II's own heparin binding site, and is displaced in the presence of heparin.[109,112] In the process, this tail becomes available for binding to the fibrinogen recognition exosite of thrombin (Fig. 6, see next page). Heparin (or dermatan sulphate) therefore plays a dual role in promoting thrombin inhibition by heparin cofactor II. The numerous exosite interactions allow the binding of an unfavourable P1 residue, and ensure that only thrombin is inhibited due to its unique fibrinogen recognition exosite.

VI. SUMMARY

The wealth of structural information now available for thrombin, its precursors, it substrates and its inhibitors allows us to understand the many roles of thrombin. α-Thrombin exhibits an unusually deep and narrow active site cleft, formed by loop insertions characteristic of thrombin. This canyon structure is one of the prime causes for the narrow specificity of thrombin. As a result of the conjunction of amino acid residues of like properties, such as charge or hydrophobicity, thrombin can be divided up into a number of functional regions. The apposition of the active site to a hydrophobic pocket (the apolar binding site) on one side and a basic patch (the fibrinogen recognition exosite) on the other side allows for a fine tuning of enzymatic activity, as seen for fibrinogen. These two sites also are used optimally by the leech-derived inhibitor hirudin, allowing the very tight binding observed; thrombin inhibition is effected by blocking access to the active site. Interactions with antithrombin III are tightened with the help of heparin, which binds to a second basic site (the heparin binding site). Non-proteolytic cellular properties are attributed to the rigid insertion loop at Tyr60A.

The use of these sites by various proteins is shown schematically in Fig. 6.[17] By making numerous interactions at a large number of sites (see Fig. 5), the interaction with fibrinogen allows for highly specific recognition. Binding to the membrane bound thrombomodulin is probably via the fibrinogen recognition exosite; this could have the effect of altering the S3' site, allowing binding and cleavage (and thereby activation) of protein C.[17,26] The thrombin receptor might bind in the unprimed site similarly to protein C; however, it carries its own exosite binding region near the cleavage site. Hirudin, for which sound structural data are available, covers the active site cleft of thrombin with its N-terminal globular domain, restricting access to the catalytic residues for macromolecular substrates.[21-24] The inhibition is considerably strengthened by numerous interactions of the extended C-terminal tail with the fibrinogen recognition exosite. The

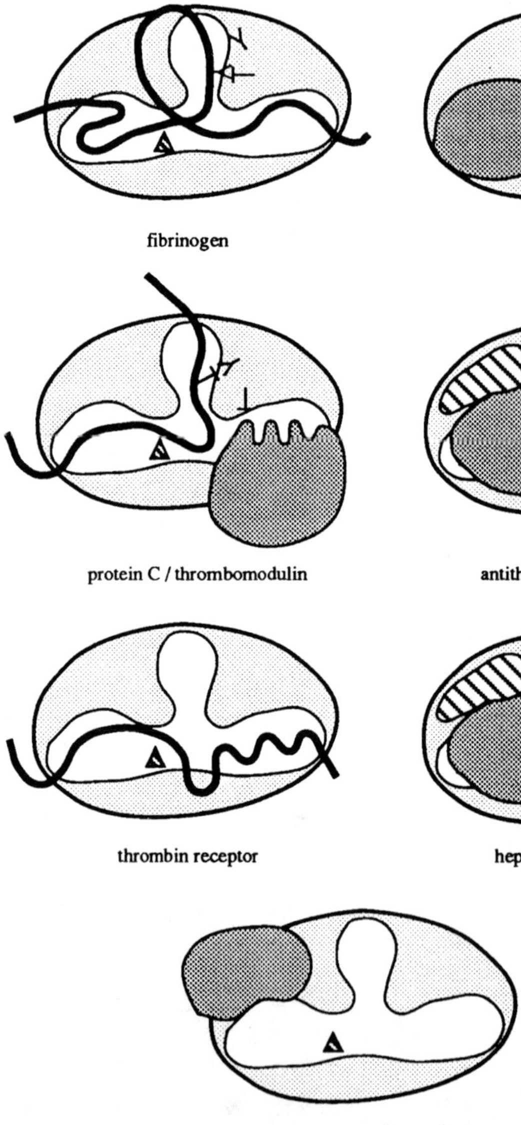

Figure 6. Schematic (and highly simplified) diagram of the interactions of α-thrombin, both observed and speculative; note that experimental data exist only for the interaction with hirudin[21-24], fibrinopeptide A[26,27], and prothrombin kringle F2.[28] The thrombin molecule corresponds to Fig. 3 in the standard orientation, with the active site in the middle (▲), the unprimed sites to the left, and the fibrinogen recognition exosite to the right (Y and T represent basic and acidic residues of the hypothetical S3' site, respectively; see Fig. 5)

modelled interaction of thrombin with α_1-proteinase inhibitor (related to antithrombin III) suggests binding of the active site loop in a canonical conformation.[90] The putative complex would bring the heparin binding sites of thrombin and antithrombin III together, allowing linkage of the components via heparin. Heparin cofactor II makes additional use of the fibrinogen recognition exosite, making up for an unfavourable hydrophobic P1 residue. The structure of the complex of prothrombin kringle F2 and thrombin show that the kringle occupies the putative heparin binding site.[28] Through the "mix-and-match" nature of interactions with the various modules of α-thrombin, this highly diverse molecule is able to participate in an overwhelming number of activities, with the high degree of specificity necessary for the fine regulation of hemostasis.

The observed rigidity of the thrombin molecule in its complexes makes thrombin ideal for structure based drug design (see ref.[17]). Thrombin can be inhibited either at the active site, at the fibrinogen recognition exosite, or at both. Structural information shows that binding at the former is enhanced by good fit of aromatic moieties to the aryl- and S2 binding sites (the apolar binding site). Binding at the fibrinogen recognition exosite is facilitated by negative charged groups. The unpredictable nature of inhibitor binding suggests that drug design should go hand in hand with crystallographic experiments.

ACKNOWLEDGEMENTS

We would like to thank Professor Robert Huber for his constant support and interest in this work, and Professor Alexander Tulinsky for fruitful collaborations. Parts of this work were supported by the Sonderforschungsbereich 207 to WB; MTS is supported by Organon International B.

REFERENCES

1. **Furie, B. and Furie, B.C.** The molecular basis of blood coagulation. *Cell* 53, 505, 1988.
2. **Vu, T.K.H., Hung, D.T., Wheaton, V.I. and Coughlin, S.R.** Molecular cloning of a functional thrombin receptor reveals a novel proteolytic mechanism of receptor activation. *Cell* 64, 1057, 1991.
3. **Rasmussen, U.B., Vouret-Craviari, V., Jallat, S., Schlesinger, Y., Pages, G., Pavirani, A., Lecocq, J-P., Pouyssegur, J. and VanObberghen-Schilling, E.** cDNA cloning and expression of

a hamster α-thrombin receptor coupled to Ca^{2+} mobilization. *FEBS Lett* 288, 123, 1991.

4. **Esmon, C.T.** The roles of protein C and thrombomodulin in the regulation of blood coagulation. *J Biol Chem* 264, 4743, 1989.
5. **Rosenberg, R.D. and Damus, P.S.** The purification and mechanism of action of human antithrombin-heparin cofactor. *J Biol Chem* 248, 6490, 1973.
6. **Tollefsen, D.M., Majerus, D.W. and Blank, M.K.** Heparin cofactor II. Purification and properties of a heparin-dependent inhibitor of thrombin in human plasma. *J Biol Chem* 257, 2162, 1982.
7. **Cunningham, D.D. and Farrell, D.H.** Thrombin interactions with cultured fibroblasts: relationship to mitogenic stimulation. *Ann NY Acad USA* 485, 240, 1986.
8. **Bjork, I. and Lindahl, V.** Mechanism of the anticoagulant action of heparin. *Mol Cell Biochem* 48, 161, 1982.
9. **Walsmann, P. and Markwardt, F.** Biochemische und pharmakologische Aspekte des Thrombininhibitors Hirudin. *Pharmazie* 36, 653, 1981.
10. **Stone, S.R. and Hofsteenge, J.** Kinetics of the inhibition of thrombin by hirudin. *Biochem* 25, 4622-4628, 1986.
11. **Dodt, J., Kohler, S. and Baici, A.** Interaction of site specific hirudin variants with α-thrombin. *FEBS Lett* 229, 87, 1988.
12. **Steiner, V., Knecht, R., Bornsen, K.O., Gassmann, E., Stone, S.R., Raschdorf, F., Schlaeppi, J.M. and Maschler, R.** Primary structure and function of novel O-glycosylated hirudins from the leech Hirudinaria manillensis. *Biochem* 31, 2294, 1992.
13. **Strube, K.H., Kroger, B., Biolajan, S., Otte, M. and Dodt, J.** Isolation, sequence analysis, and cloning of haemadin. *J Biol Chem* 268, 8590, 1993.
14. **Friedrich, T., Kroger, B., Biolajan, S., Lemaire, H.G., Hoffken, H.W., Reuschenbach, P., Otte, M. and Dodt, J.** A Kazal-type inhibitor with thrombin specificity from Rhodnius prolixus. *J Biol Chem* 268, 16216, 1993.
15. **Zingali, R.B., Jandrot-Perrus, M., Guillin, M-C. and Bon, C.** Bothrojaracin, a new thrombin inhibitor isolated from Bothrops jararaca venom: Characterization and mechanism of thrombin inhibition. *Biochem* 32, 1074, 1993.
16. **Bar-Shavit, R., Benezra, M., Sabbah, V., Bode, W. and Vlodavsky, L.** Thrombin as a multifunctional protein: induction of cell adhesion and proliferation. *Am J Respir Cell Mol Biol* 6, 123, 1992.
17. **Stubbs, M.T. and Bode, W.** A player of many parts: the spotlight falls on thrombin's structure. *Thromb Res* 69, 1, 1993.

18. **Cunningham, D.D., Pulliam, L. and Vaughan, P.J.** Protease nexin-1 and thrombin: Injury related processes in the brain. *Thromb Haemost* 70, 168, 1993.
19. **Bode, W., Mayr, I., Baumann, U., Huber, R., Stone, S.R. and Hofsteenge, J.** The refined 1.9 Å crystal structure of human α-thrombin: Interaction with D-Phe-Pro-Arg chloromethlyketone and significance of the Tyr-Pro-Pro-Trp insertion segment. *EMBO J* 8, 3467, 1989.
20. **Bode, W., Turk, D. and Karshikov, A.** The refined 1.9 Å X-ray crystal structure of D-Phe-ProArg chloromethylketone inhibited human α-thrombin. Structure analysis, overall structure, electrostatic properties, detailed active site geometry, structure-function relationships. *Protein Sci* 1, 426, 1992.
21. **Rydel, T. J., Ravichandran, K.G., Tulinsky, A., Bode, W., Huber, R., Roitsch, C., and Fenton, J.W., II.** The structure of a complex of recombinant hirudin and human α-thrombin, *Science* 249, 277, 1990.
22. **Rydel, T.J., Tulinsky, A., Bode, W. and Huber, R.** Refined structure of the hirudin-thrombin complex. *J Mol Biol* 221, 583, 1991.
23. **Grütter, M.G., Priestle, J.P., Rahuel, J., Grossenbacher, H., Bode, W., Hofsteenge, J. and Stone, S.R.** Crystal structure of the thrombin-hirudin complex: A novel mode of serine protease inhibitor. *EMBO J* 9, 2361, 1990.
24. **Vitali, J., Martin, P.D., Malkowski, M.G., Robertson, W.D., Lazar, J.B., Winant, R.C., Johnson, P.J. and Edwards, B.F.P.** The structure of a complex of bovine α-thrombin and recombinant hirudin at 2.8 Å resolution. *J Biol Chem* 267, 17670, 1992.
25. **Skrzypczak-Jankun, E., Carperos, V., Ravichandran, K.G., Tulinsky, A., Westbrook, M. and Maraganore, J.** The structure of the hirugen and hirulog 1 complexes of α-thrombin. *J Mol Biol* 221, 1379, 1991.
26. **Stubbs, M.T., Oschkinat, H., Mayr, I., Huber, R., Angliker, H., Stone, S.R. and Bode, W.** The interaction of thrombin with fibrinogen — a structural basis for its specificity. *Eur J Biochem* 206, 187, 1992.
27. **Martin, P.D., Robertson, W., Turk, D., Bode, W. and Edwards, B.F.P.** The structure of residues 7-16 of the Aα-chain of human fibrinogen bound to bovine thrombin at 2.3 Å resolution. *J Biol Chem* 267, 7911, 1992.
28. **Arni, R.K., Padmanabhan, K., Padmanabhan, K.P., Wu, T.P. and Tulinsky, A.** Structures of the non-covalent complexes of

human and bovine prothrombin fragment 2 with human PPACK-thrombin. *Biochem* 32, 4727, 1993.

29. **Bode, W., Turk, D. and Sturzebecher, J.** Geometry of binding of the benzamidine- and arginine-based inhibitors NAPAP and MQPA to human α-thrombin. X-ray crystallographic determination of the NAPAP-trypsin complex and modeling NAPAP-thrombin and MQPA-thrombin. *Eur J Biochem* 193, 175, 1990.
30. **Turk, D., Sturzebecher, J. and Bode, W.** Geometry of binding of α-tosylated piperidides of m-amidino, p-amidino- and p-guanidino phenylalanine to thrombin and trypsin. X-ray crystal structures of their trypsin complexes and modeling of their thrombin complexes. *FEBS Lett* 287, 133, 1991.
31. **Matsuzaki, T., Sasaki, C., Okumura, C. and Umeyama, H.** X-ray analysis of a thrombin inhibitor-trypsin complex. *J Biochem (Tokyo)* 105, 949, 1989.
32. **Brandstetter, H., Turk, D., Hoeffken, W., Grosse, D., Stuzebecher, J., Martin, P.D., Edwards, B.F.P. and Bode, W.** Refined 2.3 Å X-ray crystal structure of bovine thrombin complexes formed with the benzamidine- and arginine-based inhibitors NAPAP, 4-TAPAP and MQPA: A starting point for improving antithrombitics. *J Mol Biol* 4226, 1085, 1992.
33. **Banner, D.W. and Hadvary, P.** Crystallographic analysis at 3.0 Å resolution of the binding to human thrombin of four active site-directed inhibitors. *J Biol Chem* 266, 20085, 1991.
34. **Wu, T.P., Yee, V., Tulinsky, A., Chrusciel, R.A., Nakanashi, H., Shen, R., Priebe, C. and Kahn, M.** The structure of a designed peptidomimetic inhibitor complex of α-thrombin. *Protein Eng* 6, 471, 1993.
35. **Maryanoff, B.E., Qiu, X., Padmanabhan, K.P., Tulinsky, A., Almond, H.R., Jr., Andrade-Gordon, P., Greco, M.N., Kauffman, J.A., Nicolaou, K.C., Liu, A., Brungs, P.H. and Fusetani, N.** Molecular basis for the inhibition of human α-thrombin by the macrocyclic peptide cyclotheonamide A. *Proc Natl Acad Sci USA* 90, 8048, 1992.
36. **Qiu, X., Yin, M., Padmanabhan, K.P., Krstenansky, J.L. and Tulinsky, A.** Structures of thrombin complexes with a designed and a natural exosite peptide inhibitor. *J Biol Chem* 268, 20318, 1993.
37. **Padmanabhan, K., Padmanabhan, K.P., Ferrara, J.D., Sadler, J.E. and Tulinsky, A.** The structure of α-thrombin inhibited by a 15-mer single stranded DNA aptamer. *J Biol Chem* 268, 17651, 1993.
38. **Qiu, X., Padmanabhan, K., Carperos, V.E., Tulinsky, A., Kline,**

T., Maraganore, J.M. and Fenton, J.W., II. The structure of the hirulog3-thrombin complex and the nature of the S' subsites of substrates and inhibitors. *Biochem* 31, 11689, 1992.

39. **Zdanov, A., Wu, S., DiMaio, J., Konishi, Y., Li, Y., Wu, X., Edwards, B.F.P., Martin, P.D. and Cygler, M.** Crystal structure of the complex of human α-thrombin and nonhydrolyzable bifunctional inhibitors, hirutonin-2 and hirutonin-6. *Proteins: Structure, Function and Genetics* 17, 252, 1993.
40. **Priestle, J.P., Rahuel, J., Rink, H., Tones, M. and Grütter, M.G.** Changes in interactions in complexes of hirudin derivatives and human α-thrombin due to different crystal forms. *Protein Sci* 2, 1630, 1993.
41. **Seshadri, T.P., Tulinsky, A., Skrzypczak-Jankun, E. and Park, C.H.** Structure of bovine prothrombin fragment 1 refined at 2.25 Å resolution. *J Mol Biol* 220, 481, 1991.
42. **Soriano-Garcia, M., Padmanabhan, K., deVos, A.M. and Tulinsky, A.** The Ca^{2+} ion and membrane binding structure of the Gla domain of Ca-prothrombin fragment 1. *Biochem* 31, 2554, 1992.
43. **Bode, W. and Huber, R.** Natural protein proteinase inhibitors and their interaction with proteinases. *Eur J Biochem* 204, 433, 1992.
44. **Padmanabhan, K., Padmanabhan, K.P., Tulinsky, A., Park, C.H., Bode, W., Huber, R., Blankenship, D.T., Cardin, A.D. and Kisiel, W.** Structure of human des(1-45) Factor Xa at 2.2 Å resolution. *J Mol Biol* 232, 947-966, 1993.
45. **Magnusson, S.** Thrombin and prothrombin. In: *Enzymes* P.D. Boyer (ed), Academic Press, New York and London, Vol. 3, 1971, pp 277.
46. **Tracy, P.B., Nesheim, M.E. and Mann, K.G.** Coordinate binding of factor Va and factor Xa to the unstimulated platelet. *J Biol Chem* 256, 743, 1981.
47. **Mann, K.G., Jenny, R.J. and Krishnaswamy, S.** Cofactor proteins in the assembly and expression of blood clotting enzyme complexes. *Ann Rev Biochem* 57, 915.
48. **Pryzdial, E.L.G. and Mann, K.G.** The association of coagulation factor Xa and factor Va. *J Biol Chem* 266, 8969, 1991.
49. **Tulinsky, A.** The structure of domains of blood proteins. *Thromb Haemost* 66, 16, 1991.
50. **Degen, S.J.F., MacGillivray, R.T.A. and Davie, E.W.** Characterization of the complementary deoxyribonucleic acid and gene coding for human prothrombin. *Biochemistry* 87, 2087, 1983.
51. **Schechter, I. and Berger, A.** On the size of the active site in

proteases. I Papain *Biochem Biophys Res Commun* 27, 157, 1967.

52. **Berliner, L.J. and Shen, Y.Y.L.** Physical evidence for an apolar binding site near the catalytic center of human α-thrombin. *Biochem* 16, 4622, 1977.
53. **Fenton, J.W., II, Zabinski, M.P., Hsieh, K. and Wilner, G.D.** Thrombin non-covalent protein binding and fibrin(ogen) recognition. *Thromb Haemost* 46, 177, 1981.
54. **Banfield, D.K. and MacGillivray, R.T.A.** Partial characterization of vertebrate prothrombin cDNAs: amplification and sequence analysis of the B chain of thrombin from nine different species. *Proc Natl Acad Sci USA* 89, 2779, 1992.
55. **LeBonniec, B.F., Guinto, E.R., MacGillivray, R.T.A., Stone, S.R. and Esmon, C.T.** The role of thrombin's Tyr-Pro-Pro-Trp motif in the interaction with fibrinogen, thrombomodulin, protein C, antithrombin III, and the Kunitz inhibitors. *J Biol Chem* 268, 19055, 1993.
56. **LeBonniec, B.F., Guinto, G.R. and Esmon, C.T.** Interaction of thrombin des-ETW with antithrombin III, the Kunitz inhibitors, thrombomodulin and protein C. Structural link between the autolysis loop and the Tyr-Pro-Pro-Trp insertion of thrombin. *J Biol Chem* 267, 19341, 1992.
57. **Karshikov, A.D., Engh, R., Bode, W. and Atanasov, B.P.** Electrostatic interactions in proteins: Calculations of the electrostatic term of free energy and the electrostatic potential field. *Eur Biophys J* 17, 287, 1989.
58. **Church, F.C., Pratt, C.W., Noyes, C.M., Kalayanamit, T., Sherril, G.B., Tobin, R.B. and Meade, B.** Structural and functional properties of human α-thrombin, phosphopyridoxylated α-thrombin and γ_T-thrombin. Identification of lysyl residues in α-thrombin that are critical for heparin and fibrin(ogen) interactions. *J Biol Chem* 264, 18419, 1989.
59. **Gan, Z.R., Li, Y., Chen, Z., Lewis, S.D. and Shafer, J.A.** Identification of basic amino acid residues in thrombin essential for heparin-catalyzed inactivation by antithrombin. *J Biol Chem* 269, 1301, 1994.
60. **Dettner, C. and Shaw, E.** Inactivation of trypsin-like enzymes with peptides of arginine chloromethyl ketone. *Method Enzymol* 80, 826, 1981.
61. **Ni, F., Ripoli, D.R., Martin, P.D. and Edwards, B.F.P.** Solution structure of a platelet receptor peptide bound to bovine α-thrombin. *Biochem* 31, 11551, 1992.
62. **Svendsen, L., Blomback, B., Blomback, M. and Olsson, P.I.**

Synthetic chromogenic substrates for determination of trypsin, thrombin and thrombin-like enzymes. *Thromb Res* 1, 267, 1972.

63. **Karshikov, A., Bode, W., Tulinsky, A. and Stone, S.R.** Electrostatic interactions in the association of proteins: an analysis of the thrombin-hirudin complex. *Protein Sci* 1, 727, 1992.
64. **Betz, A., Hofsteenge, J. and Stone, S.R.** Role of interactions involving C-terminal nonpolar residues of hirudin in the formation of the thrombin-hirudin complex. *Biochem* 30, 9848, 1991.
65. **Betz, A., Hofsteenge, J. and Stone, S.R.** Ionic interactions in the formation of the thrombin-hirudin complex. *Biochem J* 275, 801, 1991.
66. **White, G.C., Lundblad, R.L. and Griffith, M.J.** Structure-function relations in platelet-thrombin reactins. *J Biol Chem* 256, 1763, 1981.
67. **Griffith, M.J., Kingdon, H.S. and Lundblad, R.L.** The interaction of heparin with human α-thrombin: Effect on the hydrolysis of anilide tripeptide substrates. *Arch Biochem Biophys* 195, 378, 1979.
68. **Bourin, M-C. and Lindahl, U.** Glycosaminoglycans and the regulation of blood coagulation. *Biochem J* 289, 313, 1993.
69. **Walker, F.J. and Esmon, C.T.** The effect of prothrombin fragment 2 on the inhibition of thrombin by antithrombin III. *J Biol Chem* 254, 5618, 1979.
70. **Bourin, M-C., Ohlin, A-K., Lane, D.A., Stenflo, J. and Lindahl, U.** Relationship between anticoagulant activities and polyanionic properties of rabbit thrombomodulin. *J Biol Chem* 263, 8044, 1988.
71. **Olson, T.A., Sonder, S.A. Wilner, G.D. and Fenton, J.W., II.** Heparin binding in proximity to the catalytic site of human α-thrombin. *Ann NY Acad Sci* 485, 96, 1986.
72. **Ofosu, F.A., Hirsh J., Esmon, C.T., Modi, G.J., Smith, L.M., Anvari, N., Buchanan, M.R., Fenton, J.W., II. and Blajchman, M.A.** Unfractionated heparin inhibits thrombin-catalysed amplification reactions of coagulation more efficiently than those catalysed by Factor Xa. *Biochem J* 257, 143, 1989.
73. **Hageman, T.C. and Scheraga, H.A.** Mechanism of action of thrombin on fibrinogen; Reaction of the N-terminal CNBR fragment from the Aα chain of human fibrinogen with bovine thrombin. *Arch Biochem Biophys* 164, 707, 1974.
74. **Hogg, D.H. and Blomback, B.** The specificity of the fibrinogen-thrombin interaction. *Thromb Res* 5, 685, 1974.
75. **Binnie, C.G. and Lord, S.T.** The fibrinogen sequences that interact with thrombin. *Blood* 81, 3186, 1993.

76. **Ni, F., Meinwald, Y.C., Vasquez, M. and Scheraga, H.A.** High resolution NMR studies of fibrinogen-like peptides in solution structure of a thrombin-bound peptide corresponding to residues 7-16 of the Aα chain of human fibrinogen. *Biochem* 28, 3094, 1989.
77. **Lord, S.T., Byrd, P.A., Hede, K.L., Wei, C. and Colby, T.J.** Analysis of fibrinogen Aα-fusion proteins. Mutants which inhibit thrombin equivalently are not equally good substrates. *J Biol Chem* 265, 838, 1990.
78. **Naski, M.C., Fenton, J.W., II., Maraganore, J.M., Olson, S.T. and Shafer, J.A.** The COOH-terminal domain of hirudin. An exosite-directed competitive inhibitor of the action of α-thrombin on fibrinogen. *J Biol Chem* 265, 13484, 1990.
79. **Schmitz, T., Rothe, M. and Dodt, J.** Mechanism of the inhibition of α-thrombin by hirudin-derived fragments hirudin (1-47) and hirudin (45-65). *Eur J Biochem* 195, 251, 1991.
80. **Binnie, C.G. and Lord, S.T.** A synthetic analog of fibrinogen α27-50 is an inhibitor of thrombin. *Thromb Haemost* 65, 615, 1991.
81. **Naski, M.C., Lorand, L. and Shafer, J.A.** Characterization of the kinetic pathway for fibrin promotion of α-thrombin-catalyzed activation of plasma factor XIII. *Biochem* 30, 934, 1991.
82. **Dodt, J., Seemuller, V., Maschler, R. and Fritz, H.** The complete covalent structure of hirudin. Localization of the disulphide bonds. *Biol Chem Hoppe-Seyler* 366, 379, 1985.
83. **Folkers, P.J.M., Clore, G.M., Driscoll, P.C., Dodt, J., Kihler, S. and Gronenborn, A.M.** Solution structure of recombinant hirudin and the Lys-47-Glu mutant: A nuclear magnetic resonance and hybrid distance geometry-dynamical simulated annealing study. *Biochem* 28, 2601, 1989.
84. **Haruyama, H. and Wuthrich, K.** The conformation of recombinant disulfatohirudin in aqueous solution determined by nuclear magnetic resonance. *Biochem* 28, 4301, 1989.
85. **Betz, A., Hofsteenge, J. and Stone, S.R.** Interaction of the N-terminal region of hirudin with the active-site cleft of thrombin. *Biochem* 31, 4557, 1992.
86. **Winant, R.C., Lazar, J.B. and Johnson, P.H.** Chemical modifications and amino acid substitutions in recombinant hirudin that increase hirudin-thrombin affinity. *Biochem* 30, 1271, 1991.
87. **Fenton, J.W., II, Ofosu, F.A., Moon, D.G. and Maraganore, J.M.** Thrombin structure and function: why thrombin is the primary target for antithrombotics. *Blood Coag Fibrin* 2, 69, 1991.
88. **Owen, M.C., Brennan, S.O., Lewis, J.H. and Carrell, R.W.**

Mutation of antitrypsin to antithrombin. Antitrypsin Pittsburgh (358Met-Arg), a fatal bleeding disorder. *N Engl J Med* 309, 694, 1983.

89. **Huber, R. and Carrell, R.W.** Implications of the three-dimensional structure of α_1-antitrypsin for structure and function of serpins. *Biochem* 28, 8951, 1989.
90. **Engh, R.A., Schulze, A.J., Huber, R. and Bode, W.** Serpin structures. *Behring Inst Mitt* 93, 1993.
91. **Bruch, M., Weiss, V. and Engel, J.** Plasma serine proteinase inhibitors (serpins) exhibit major conformational changes and a large increase in conformational stability upon cleavage at their reactive sites. *J Biol Chem* 263, 16626, 1988.
92. **Carrell, R.W. and Owen, M.C.** Plakalbumin, α_1-antitrypsin, antithrombin and the mechanism of inflammatory thrombosis. *Nature* 4317, 730, 1989.
93. **Engh, R.A., Wright, H.T. and Huber, R.** Modelling the intact form of the α_1-proteinase inhibitor. *Protein Eng* 3, 346, 1990.
94. **Lobermann, H., Tokuoka, R., Deisenhofer, J. and Huber, R.** Human α_1-proteinase inhibitor. Crystal structure analysis of two crystal modifications, molecular model and preliminary analysis of the implications for function. *J Mol Biol* 177, 531, 1984.
95. **Engh, R., Lobermann, H., Schneider, M., Wiegand, G., Huber, R. and Laurell, C.B.** The S variant of human α_1-antitrypsin, structure and implications for function and metabolism. *Protein Eng* 2, 407, 1989.
96. **Wright, H.T., Qian, H.X. and Huber R.** Crystal structure of plakalbumin, a proteolytically nicked form of ovalbumin. Its relationship to the structure of cleaved α_1-proteinase inhibitor. *J Mol Biol* 213, 513, 1990.
97. **Stein, P.E., Leslie, A.G.W., Finch, J.T., Turnell, W.G., McLaughlin, P.J. and Carrell, R.W.** Crystal structure of ovalbumin as a model for the reactive centre of serpins. *Nature* 347, 99, 1990.
98. **Baumann, U., Huber, R., Bode, W., Grosse, D., Lesjak, M. and Laurell, C.B.** Crystal structure of cleaved human α_1-antichymotrypsin at 2.71 Å resolution and its comparison with other serpins. *J Mol Biol* 218, 595, 1991.
99. **Baumann, U., Bode, W., Huber, R., Travis, J. and Potempa, J.** Crystal structure of cleaved equine leukocyte elastase inhibitor determined at 1.95 Å resolution. *J Mol Biol* 226, 1207, 1992.
100. **Mottonen, J., Strand, A., Symersky, J., Sweet, R.M., Danley, D.E., Geoghegan, K.F., Gerard, R.D. and Goldsmith, E.J.** Structural basis of latency in plasminogen-activator inhibitor-1. *Nature* 355, 270, 1992.

101. **Mourey, L., Samama, J-L., Delarue, M., Petitou, M., Choay, J. and Moras, D.** Crystal structure of cleaved bovine antithrombin III at 3.2 Å resolution. *J Mol Biol* 232, 223, 1993.
102. **Wei, A., Rubin, H., Cooperman, B.S. and Christianson, D.W.** Crystal structure of an uncleaved serpin reveals the conformation of an inhibitory reactive loop. *Nature Struct Biol*, In Press.
103. **Schreuder, H.A., deBoer, B., Dijkema, R., Mulders, J., Theunissen, H.J.M., Grootenhuis, P.D.J. and Hol, W.G.J.** Crystal structure of a complex between intact and cleaved human antithrombin III as a model for serpin-proteinase interaction. *Nature Struct Biol* 1, 48, 1994.
104. **Schulze, A.J., Huber, R., Degryse, E., Speck, D. and Bischoff, R.** Inhibitory activity and conformational transition of α_1-proteinase inhibitor variants. *Eur J Biochem* 202, 1147, 1991.
105. **Skriver, K., Wikoff, W.R., Patston, P.A., Tausk, F., Schapira, M., Kaplan, A.P. and Bock, S.C.** Substitution properties of C1 inhibition Ma (Alanine 434-Glutamic acid). General and structural evidence suggesting that the P12-region contains critical determinants of serine protease inhibitor inhibitor/substrate status. *J Biol Chem* 266, 9216, 1991.
106. **Schulze, A.J., Baumann, U., Knof, S., Jaeger, E., Huber, R. and Laurell, C.B.** Structural transition of α_1-antitrypsin by a peptide sequentially similar to ß-strand s4A. *Eur J Biochem* 194, 51, 1990.
107. **Bjork, I., Ylinenjarvi, K., Olson, S.T. and Bock, P.E.** Conversion of antithrombin from an inhibitor of thrombin to a substrate with reduced heparin affinity and enhanced conformational stability by binding of a tetradecapeptide corresponding to the P1 to P14 region of the putative reactive bond loop of the inhibitor. *J Biol Chem* 267, 1976, 1992.
108. **Schulze, A.J., Frohnert, P.W., Engh, R.A. and Huber, R.** Evidence for the extent of insertion of the active site loop of intact α_1-proteinase inhibitor in ß-sheet A. *Biochem* 31, 7560, 1992.
109. **VanDeerlin, V.M.D. and Tollefsen, D.M.** The N-terminal acidic domain of heparin cofactor II mediates the inhibition of α-thrombin in the presence of glycosaminoglycans. *J Biol Chem* 266, 20223, 1991.
110. **Rogers, S.J., Pratt, C.W., Whinna, H.C. and Church, F.C.** Role of thrombin exosites in inhibition by heparin cofactor II. *J Biol Chem* 267, 3613, 1992.
111. **Leong, L., Henriksen, R.A., Kermode, J.C., Rittenhouse, S.E. and Tracy, P.B.** The thrombin high affinity binding site on platelets is a negative regulator of thrombin-induced platelet

activation. Structure-function studies using two mutant thrombins, Quick 1 and Quick II. *Biochem* 31, 2567, 1992.
112. **Ragg, H., Ulshofer, T. and Gerewitz, J.** On the activation of human Leuserpin-2, a thrombin inhibitor, by glycosaminoglycans. *J Biol Chem* 265, 5211, 1990.
113. **Ragg, H., Ulshofer, T. and Gerewitz, J.** Glycosaminoglycan-mediated Leuserpin-2/thrombin interaction. Structure function relationships. *J Biol Chem* 265, 22386, 1990.
114. **Pomerantz, M.W. and Owen, W.G.** A catalytic role for heparin. Evidence for a ternary complex of heparin cofactor thrombin and heparin. *Biochim Biophys Acta* 535, 66, 1978.
115. **Griffith, M.J.** Kinetics of the heparin-enhanced antithrombin III/thrombin reaction. Evidence for a template model for the mechanism of action of heparin. *J Biol Chem* 257, 7360, 1982.
116. **Nesheim, M.E.** A simple rate law that describes the kinetics of the heparin-catalyzed reaction between antithrombin III and thrombin. *J Biol Chem* 258, 1408, 1983.

Chapter 3

DEVELOPMENT AND RATIONALE FOR THE USE OF LOW MOLECULAR WEIGHT HEPARINS IN THE PREVENTION AND TREATMENT OF VENOUS THROMBOSIS

Jacques R. Leclerc

I. INTRODUCTION

Thrombin is one of the key enzymes of blood coagulation. It exerts multiple effects on blood coagulation, including the conversion of fibrinogen into fibrin, Factor XIII activation, platelet activation and the activation of the protein C pathway. Thrombin also exerts positive feedback reactions that amplify the coagulation mechanisms, i.e. the retrograde activation of Factors V to Va and VIII to VIIIa. There is increasing evidence that the main effect of heparin in human plasma is to increase the rate of thrombin inhibition.[1] Low molecular weight heparins exhibit a greater anti-Factor Xa than an anti-thrombin activity. Despite their reduced anti-thrombin activity, low molecular weight heparins are very good antithrombotic agents with proven efficacy in clinical studies. In this chapter, the rationale for the use of low molecular weight heparins in the prevention and treatment of venous thromboembolic disease is reviewed. The differential effects of unfractionated heparin and low molecular weight heparins on blood coagulation provide us with new insights on the physiology of hemostasis and the chemistry of glycosaminoglycans in general.

II. UNFRACTIONATED HEPARIN

A. HISTORY

Heparin was discovered in 1916 by Jay McLean[2],a medical student at Johns Hopkins University. During his one-year research project, McLean was given the task of investigating whether dog liver extracts would promote blood coagulation. Much to his dismay, he found quite the contrary: his canine liver extracts delayed blood coagulation. This anticoagulant substance was named heparin (from the Greek word hepar meaning liver) by William Howell in 1918. It took several years before the importance of McLean's fortuitous discovery was fully appreciated. His discovery opened new avenues in the treatment of thromboembolic disorders and made possible the development of cardiac surgery and hemodialysis. There are few examples in medicine of major breakthrough discoveries that occurred within a one-year time frame. Despite its discovery nearly 80 years

0-8493-7649-1/95/$0.00+$.50

ago, the structure and mechanism of action of heparin is still an area of active investigation by several laboratories worldwide.[1,3,4] Heparin is the most widely used drug in the prevention and treatment of thrombotic disorders. Approximately 33 metric tons, representing 500 million doses of heparin, are used worldwide each year. The main uses of unfractionated heparin are shown in Table 1. Despite its widespread use, heparin has a number of limitations which have provided incentives for the development of newer heparins. These limitations of heparin are based on its pharmacokinetic, hemostatic and clinical properties (Table 2).

B. LIMITATIONS OF UNFRACTIONATED HEPARIN

1. Pharmacokinetics

The pharmacokinetic profile of unfractionated heparin is complex and not completely understood.[5-8] Studies performed in healthy volunteers have shown that the half-life of intravenous heparin, as measured by its anticoagulant activity, increases with the dose administered.[8] For example, the clearance half-lives of bolus doses of heparin of 100, 200 and 400 U/kg are 60, 90 and 120 minutes, respectively.[9] Similarly, the half-life of subcutaneous heparin increases with the dose administered. This dose relationship of heparin half-life may explain the variability in time and dose required to achieve a steady-state therapeutic anticoagulation among individuals. It may also explain the limited bioavailability of heparin at low doses. The importance of achieving rapidly a therapeutic level of anticoagulation in patients with venous thrombosis has been highlighted in a randomized trial comparing continuous intravenous heparin with an adjusted-dose subcutaneous regimen.[10] The results showed that the subcutaneous regimen failed to achieve a therapeutic anticoagulant response in the majority of patients. This resulted in a high incidence (19%) of recurrent venous thromboembolism. In contrast, the intravenous regimen yielded a therapeutic response in the majority of patients and a lower rate of recurrent events (5%). The odds of recurrence in patients who failed to achieve therapeutic anticoagulation were 15:1.[3]

Heparin clearance appears mediated by two main mechanisms: 1) saturable and 2) non-saturable.[6,8] The saturable mechanism is probably due to heparin binding to the endothelium[11] and the reticuloendothelial system[12] as well as to plasma proteins other than antithrombin III (ATIII), including von Willebrand Factor (vWF)[13], platelet factor-4[14], histidine-rich glycoprotein[15], fibronectin and vitronectin.[16] Heparin binding to these other proteins may explain the well-known phenomenon of heparin resistance, i.e. failure of therapeutic heparin to prolong the activated partial thromboplastin

Table 1
Clinical Uses of Unfractionated Heparin

Venous Thromboembolism
- Prevention of venous thromboembolism in high risk patients
- Treatment of acute pulmonary embolism (PE) or deep vein thrombosis (DVT)

Cardiac disease
- Unstable angina
- Prevention of mural thrombus formation after myocardial infarction
- After thrombolytic therapy
- Treatment of cardioembolic stroke

During Certain Procedures
- Coronary or peripheral leg angioplasty
- Cardiac catheterization
- Vascular bypass graft surgery
- Cardiac bypass surgery
- Hemodialysis

Prevention of Catheter Thrombosis

Table 2
Limitations of Unfractionated Heparin

Pharmacokinetic
- Half-life influenced by dose administered
- Heparin binds to plasma proteins and the endothelium, resulting in low bioavailability at low doses, variability in dose response and heparin resistance in certain patients

Hemostatic
- Interferes with platelet function
- Increases vessel wall permeability

Clinical
- Requires careful laboratory monitoring when given in therapeutic doses
- Incidence of major hemorrhage of 2-8% when given in therapeutic doses
- May cause thrombocytopenia
- Prolonged use may cause osteoporosis
- High incidence of residual proximal deep vein thrombosis after major orthopedic surgery of the lower limb

time (aPTT) despite a heparin dose that appears adequate. Heparin binding to these proteins, some of which are acute phase reactants, reduces the concentration available to bind ATIII and, therefore, its anticoagulant activity. Young and colleagues[17] investigated the effect of protein binding on the anticoagulant activity of heparin, using a chemically modified heparin that did not bind to ATIII (low affinity heparin). When plasma from patients with venous thrombosis was spiked with heparin, the recovery of anti-Factor Xa activity increased markedly after adding an excess of low affinity heparin. The addition of low affinity heparin displaced the large proportion of heparin that had been reversibly bound by the plasma proteins other than ATIII. An even higher recovery of anti-Factor Xa activity was observed when similar experiments were performed using samples from patients with venous thrombosis who exhibited heparin resistance. The phenomenon of heparin resistance sometimes encountered in sick patients may be due to heparin binding to acute phase reactants, thus decreasing its bioavailability. One of those acute phase reactants, Factor VIII:C/vWF, has a profound effect on the aPTT. High level of Factor VIII:C shortens the aPTT. The only reliable mean of assessing heparin therapy in patients whose aPTT remains sub-therapeutic despite a heparin dose that appears adequate, i.e. ≥40,000 U/day, is to perform a plasma heparin assay. The therapeutic range is 0.4-0.5 U/ml when measured by the protamine sulfate neutralization method.[18] This corresponds to a range of 0.3-0.6 IU/ml by the anti-Factor Xa method. Unfortunately, heparin assays are expensive and not routinely available in many hospital laboratories.

Renal clearance appears to account for the non-saturable, linear elimination of heparin.[6] Renal elimination occurs following heparin desulfation by the liver and spleen.[7]

2. Hemostatic

Heparin induces a primary hemostatic defect that may, in turn, contribute to its hemorrhagic potential. Heparin prolongs the bleeding time in man.[19] The primary hemostatic defect of heparin has been ascribed to the inhibition of collagen- and ristocetin-induced platelet aggregation[4], interference with vWF function[13] and an increase in vessel wall permeability.[20] Fernandez and co-workers[21] observed a relationship between the inhibition of collagen-induced platelet aggregation by heparin and microvascular bleeding in rabbits.

3. Clinical Complications of Heparin

The variation in heparin dose requirements to achieve a steady state of therapeutic anticoagulation, coupled with the recognition that the aPTT must be maintained within a therapeutic range of 2 to 2 1/2 times the laboratory control value, provides the need for careful laboratory monitoring of patients who are therapeutically anticoagulated. The need for laboratory monitoring is one of the factors that precludes the ambulatory treatment of patients with acute deep vein thrombosis (DVT). There is a strong relationship between the clinical effectiveness of unfractionated heparin and the anticoagulant effect achieved. For example, Turpie and co-workers[22] conducted a randomized trial comparing two intensities of subcutaneous heparin for the prevention of mural thrombus formation in patients with anterior myocardial infarction. Sub-group analysis of this study shows a relative risk of mural thrombus formation of 22 for patients who failed to achieve a therapeutic level of anticoagulation.[3] Nomograms of heparin administration have been developed to minimize the risk of sub-therapeutic anticoagulation[23-25] but they do not eliminate entirely the cost and inconvenience of heparin monitoring. The recognition that there is significant variability in heparin responsiveness among the various commercial aPTT reagents *in vitro* and the ensuing need that each laboratory must establish its own dose relationship, further complicate the logistics of laboratory monitoring.

Hemorrhage is the most common complication of heparin administration. Contemporary studies of patients treated for venous thromboembolism indicate an incidence of major bleeding ranging from 2-8%. The consequences of major hemorrhage are not negligible, particularly when it results in a prolonged hospital stay or leads to therapeutic interventions such as the administration of blood products (which have the inherent risk of transmitting blood-borne infections).

Heparin-induced thrombocytopenia is another serious complication which occurs in up to 5% of patients who receive therapeutic doses of heparin.[26] It is thought to be due to a heparin-dependent IgG antibody that activates platelets. Heparin-induced thrombocytopenia usually develops after the fifth day of heparin therapy but may occur earlier with prior heparin sensitization. It may also develop after prolonged heparin use. This raises a particular concern for patients who receive long-term treatment (Table 3, see next page). The most feared complication of heparin-induced thrombocytopenia is venous or arterial thrombosis. These thromboembolic episodes are often massive, leading to significant morbidity and mortality. Leg amputation secondary to peripheral arterial occlusion, has been reported on several occasions. Pathologic examination of these thrombi has shown that they are made of platelet aggregates and are white, thus the term "white clot syndrome".[27] Heparin-induced thrombocytopenia has also been reported in patients who receive low doses of prophylactic heparin and with "tiny" heparin doses to prevent catheter thrombosis, but its incidence is less well known in these settings. Warkentin and co-workers[28] reported a 3% incidence of heparin-induced thrombocytopenia in patients receiving unfractionated heparin for the prevention of venous thromboembolism after hip arthroplasty.

Long-term heparin administration may cause osteoporosis. Selected indications for long-term heparin administration are listed in Table 3. Griffith and co-workers[29] found a high incidence of symptomatic osteoporosis in patients who received more than 15,000 units daily for more than 6 months. DeSwiet and colleagues[30] found that all patients receiving more than 20,000 units daily for more than 20 weeks during pregnancy showed significant bone thinning. *In vitro*, heparin can enhance bone resorption and inhibit bone cell replication and collagen synthesis.[31] More recently, Ginsberg and colleagues[32]

Table 3
Selected Indications for Long-term Heparin Administration

Treatment of acute venous thromboembolism during pregnancy
Prophylaxis of venous thromboembolism during pregnancy in high risk patients, e.g. previous thromboembolic episode, thrombophilic state
Prevention of arterial thromboembolism during pregnancy in patients with mechanical prosthetic valves
Recurrent thromboembolism despite therapeutic oral anticoagulation
Oral anticoagulants malabsorption, e.g. short bowel syndrome
Need for long-term anticoagulation in patients with no venous access

reported the results of a case control study showing a higher incidence of osteopenia, measured by photon densitometry, in premenopausal women previously treated with long-term heparin compared to a control group of women matched for age, parity and never receiving heparin. On the other hand, none of the women treated with heparin developed symptomatic fractures. Heparin associated osteopenia appears to be reversible.[33]

Low dose subcutaneous heparin is a time honoured thromboprophylactic method in high risk patients. While this method has provided satisfactory results in major abdominal surgery, it remains sub-optimal in such high risk thrombogenic situations as major orthopedic surgery for the lower extremity or surgery for malignant disease. Meta-analysis of studies of low dose heparin prophylaxis in patients undergoing major orthopedic surgery have shown an overall risk reduction of 50%, corresponding to an absolute rate of residual DVT of approximately 20%.[34] However, the rate of residual proximal vein thrombosis remains unacceptably high, at approximately 15%. These results are disturbing, considering that fatal pulmonary embolism (PE) usually originates from proximal vein thrombosis.

III. LOW MOLECULAR WEIGHT HEPARINS

A. HISTORY

The development of the low molecular weight heparins was guided by the desire to obtain more effective and safer antithrombotic agents, with enhanced antithrombotic properties but without increasing the hemorrhagic risk. The studies performed during the 1970's and later have demonstrated the efficacy and safety of low dose heparin for preventing venous thromboembolism after major surgery. These studies raised the hypothesis that heparin may retain antithrombotic properties despite plasma levels that were very low or unmeasurable. In 1976, studies by Andersson and co-workers[35] and Johnson and associates[36] reported that low molecular weight heparin fractions obtained by gel chromatography had a lesser effect on the aPTT while retaining their ability to catalyze Factor Xa inhibition. These results were encouraging, given the then current hypothesis that the antithrombotic effect of heparin was related mainly to its anti-Factor Xa activity and the prohemorrhagic effect to its anticoagulant (i.e. antithrombin activity).[37] In 1982, Carter and colleagues [38] reported that for an equivalent antithrombotic effect, low molecular weight heparins produced less microvascular bleeding in the rabbit than unfractionated heparin. Clinical trials conducted in the 1980's and early 1990's demonstrated the efficacy and safety of low molecular weight heparins for preventing venous thromboembolism in general surgical and orthopedic patients and in the treatment of acute DVT. The quality of these randomized trials is almost unprecedented since most incorporated strong methodological features in their design, i.e. double blind, comparability of groups shown, stratification according to major confounding factors, proper randomization method, objective and blind interpretation of outcomes, the use of clinically relevant outcomes, and adequate statistical power. Low molecular weight heparin was approved for preventing venous thromboembolism in orthopedic patients in Canada and in the United States in 1993.

B. BIOPHYSICAL PROPERTIES

Most commercial grade heparins in North America are obtained from porcine intestinal mucosa. Heparin is a highly negative-charged, sulfated mucopolysaccharide that belongs to the family of the glycosaminoglycans. Other related compounds include dermatan sulfate, chrondroitin-4-sulfate, chondroitin-6-sulfate and heparan sulfate. Heparin is a heterogenous mixture of mucopolysaccharide chains ranging in molecular weight from 5,000 to 30,000 and with an average molecular weight of 12,000 to 15,000. Low molecular weight heparins are obtained from heparin by either chemical or enzymatic depolymerization. Low molecular weight heparins also contain a polydisperse mixture of chains ranging in molecular weight from 2,000 to 8,000 molecular weight and with an average molecular weight between 4,000 to 6,500. Thus, low molecular weight heparins are approximately one third that of unfractionated heparin. The biologic activities of both unfractionated and low molecular weight heparin are measured against international standards that have been established for each product. There are differences among the various low molecular weight fractions *in vitro* (Table 4, see page 60). However, the clinical significance of these *in vitro* differences is unknown. A unique product, lomoparan, is a heparinoid that contains a mixture of dermatan sulfate, heparan sulfate and chondroitin sulfates.

Table 4
Characteristics of Various Low Molecular Weight Heparins

	Anti-Xa to Anti-IIa Ratio	Molecular Weight (range)	Plasma Half-Life (min)	Recommended Dose		
				General Surgery	Orthopedic Surgery	Treatment
Enoxaparine	2.7:1	4,500 (3,000-8,000)	129-180	1,600 U s/c OD	3,200 U s/c OD or 2,400 U s/c BID	5,600 U s/c BID*
Fragmin	2.0:1	5,000 (2,000-9,000)	119-139	2,500 U s/c	2,500 U s/c BID or 5,000 U s/c OD	8,400 U s/c BID*
Fraxiparine	3.2:1	4,500 (2,000-8,000)	132-162	7,500 U s/c OD		31,500 U s/c OD*
Logiparin&	1.9:1	4,500 (3,000-6,000)	111	3,500 U s/c OD	50 U/kg s/c OD	12,500 s/c OD*
RD Heparin	2.0:1	6,000 (2,000-15,000)	200		50 U/kg s/c BID	
Lomoparan	20:01	6,500	1,100		750 U s/c BID	

Reproduced and adapted from Hirsh, J. and Levine, M.N. Low molecular weight heparin. Blood 79(1), 1-17, 1992.
* Weight-adjusted dose for a 70-kg patient.

IV. MECHANISM OF ACTION

Like unfractionated heparin, the anticoagulant activity of low molecular weight heparins is dependent upon a pentasaccharide sequence that binds with high affinity to ATIII. Recent studies have elucidated further the mechanism of action of both unfractionated and low molecular weight heparins.[1,39] In a purified system, the complex heparin/ATIII inactivates thrombin, Factor Xa, Factor IXa, Factor XIa and Factor XIIa.[40] In human plasma, it has been demonstrated that the mechanism of action of unfractionated heparin centers around the inhibition of thrombin: it increases the rate of thrombin inhibition.[1] It has been shown that in the plasma environment, heparin has no effect on the inhibition of the contact enzymes (Factors XIIa and XIa).[41] It has also been reported that phospholipids and Factor Va can protect Factor Xa from the actions of heparin/ATIII.[42] Thrombin exerts multiple effects on hemostasis including fibrin formation, platelet activation, protein C activation and the feedback activation of Factors V and VIII. Thrombin inhibition by the complex heparin/ATIII decreases fibrin formation and delays blood coagulation by reducing the retrograde activation of Factor V and Factor Va and Factor VIII to Factor VIIIa. These observations suggest that the antithrombotic effect of unfractionated heparin is via its ability to inhibit thrombin.[1] It has been suggested that inhibition of prothrombin activation is not due to a direct effect of heparin on prothrombinase or Factor Xa but rather to effects on thrombin inhibition and thrombin-mediated feedback reactions.[39]

There are two main mechanisms of interaction between heparin and ATIII: 1) the conformational change mechanism and 2) the template mechanism. The conformational change mechanism entails heparin-specific binding to lysine residues in ATIII which increase the affinity of ATIII for the coagulation enzyme. This conformational change is necessary and sufficient for heparin to catalyze Factor Xa inhibition by ATIII. In the template mechanism, heparin acts as a template to which both ATIII and the coagulation enzyme assemble to form a ternary complex. The template mechanism operates when heparin catalyzes thrombin inhibition by ATIII. Heparin chain length has a direct impact on these two mechanisms. Heparin chains containing less than 18 sugar residues (including the high affinity pentasaccharide unit) can only operate via the conformation mechanism. Only chains that contain both the pentasaccharide units and a total of 18 or more sugar residues can operate by the template mechanism. These observations may explain why low molecular weight heparins exhibit higher anti-Factor Xa to anti-thrombin activity ratios than unfractionated heparin since they contain a preponderance of chains having less than 18 sugar residues in their pentasaccharide unit. In contrast, unfractionated heparin is a polydispersed mixture containing predominantly chains with more than 18 sugar residues. The anti-Factor Xa and anti-thrombin activities of commercial grade unfractionated heparin are approximately 160 IU/mg. The anti-Factor Xa and anti-thrombin activities of low molecular weight heparins vary among the various preparations (Table 4).

Central among the unresolved issues of unfractionated and low molecular weight heparins is their precise antithrombotic mechanism(s). Based on the observations that thrombin is the main target of heparin, one would predict that low molecular weight heparins should be weaker antithrombotic agents than unfractionated heparin. In fact, studies performed in experimental animals have shown that on a gravimetric basis, low molecular weight heparins are weaker antithrombotic agents than unfractionated heparin.[38] It has been suggested therefore that the antithrombotic properties of low molecular weight heparins are related to their pharmacokinetic properties, namely, to a higher bioavailability and a longer half-life (see below).[39] On the other hand, studies in experimental animals using a pentasaccharide fragment which inhibits only Factor Xa suggest that the anti-Factor Xa activity of low molecular weight heparins also contributes to their antithrombotic effects. It has been proposed by Yin and co-workers[37] that inhibition of Factor Xa, preventing prothrombin conversion, would provide a better anticoagulant effect than the mere inactivation of already formed thrombin.

V. ADVANTAGES OF LOW MOLECULAR WEIGHT HEPARIN

A. Pharmacokinetics

The pharmacokinetics of low molecular weight heparins differ markedly from those of unfractionated heparin. Unlike unfractionated heparin, the half-life of low molecular weight heparins is independent of the dose administered.[6,7,43] The main pharmacokinetic hallmark of low molecular weight heparins is their lower affinity for the endothelium, histidine-rich glycoprotein, vWF, platelet factor 4 and fibronectin, when compared to unfractionated heparin.[44] As a consequence, the elimination of low molecular weight heparins is mainly via the non-saturable and linear, renal elimination mechanism.[6] These pharmacokinetic properties result in a high bioavailability of low molecular weight heparins at low doses, a longer half-life and a more predictible response than unfractionated heparin. A potentially undesirable consequence of lesser protein binding is a reduced affinity of low molecular weight heparins to protamine sulfate, resulting in an incomplete neutralization of the heparin effect. On the other hand, there are experimental data indicating that protamine sulfate is an effective antidote for the bleeding side effects of low molecular weight heparin despite its inability to completely neutralize its anticoagulant activity.[45] The longer half-life of low molecular weight heparins has made possible the use of once daily prophylactic regimens in both general surgical and orthopedic patients. A once daily administration would be a definite advantage for patients requiring long-term use, e.g. during pregnancy, but this should be evaluated in properly designed studies. The high predictability of low molecular weight heparin pharmacokinetics has made possible the development of weight-adjusted treatment regimens, without the need for aPTT monitoring. The prospect of deleting the aPTT from treatment regimens confers to the low molecular weight heparins a high clinical utility since it eliminates the shortcomings of monitoring mentioned earlier and opens the avenue for treating DVT on an outpatient basis. The main differences between unfractionated heparin and low molecular weight heparin are summarized in Table 5 (see next page).

B. Hemostatic

Experimental studies have shown that at equivalent doses, low molecular weight heparins cause less microvascular bleeding than unfractionated heparin.[38] The reduced hemorrhagic effect of low molecular weight heparins has been ascribed to a lesser inhibition of platelet function[4,21,46] and a lesser increase in vessel wall permeability.[20] Unfractionated heparin has a greater inhibitory effect on both collagen- and vWF-dependent platelet aggregation than low molecular weight heparins.[4] The improved safety profile of low molecular weight heparins is a fundamental aspect of their clinical utility. As mentioned earlier, on a gravimetric basis, low molecular weight heparins are weaker antithrombotics than unfractionated heparin. This lesser antithrombotic activity of low molecular weight heparins is compensated by their higher bioavailability and long half-life. The higher plasma levels thus achieved with the low molecular weight heparins do not cause more bleeding in view of their greater safety profile.

The effect of unfractionated heparin and low molecular weight heparins on the platelet is complicated and incompletely understood. A landmark study was presented by Salzman and co-workers in 1980.[46] These authors studied various heparin fractions, separated by gel filtration or affinity for ATIII. High molecular weight fractions (average molecular weight 20,000) were more reactive with platelets than low molecular weight fractions (average molecular weight 7,000).

Table 5
Differences Between Unfractionated Heparin and Low Molecular Weight Heparin

	Unfractionated Heparin	Low Molecular Weight Heparin
Anti-Factor Xa activity	+++	+++
Anti-thrombin activity	+++	+
Platelet aggregation activity	+++	±
Microvascular bleeding in experimental animals	++	+
Antithrombotic properties	++	+
Binding to endothelium	+++	+
Binding to other proteins of hemostasis	+++	+
Absorption from subcutaneous tissue	+	+++
Half-life	Shorter	Longer
Antigenicity	++	+
Protamine neutralization	++	+

Among high molecular weight fractions, preparations of high or low ATIII affinity were equally reactive with platelets, suggesting that the pentasaccharide is not directly involved in heparin binding to platelets. On the other hand, with low molecular weight heparins, there is an inverse correlation between anticoagulant activity and platelet reactivity in platelet-rich plasma. In platelet-rich plasma depleted of ATIII, low molecular weight heparins of high and low ATIII activity reacted equally well with platelets. These results suggest that formation of a heparin/ATIII complex prevents platelet reactivity with low molecular weight heparins.

C. Thrombocytopenia

Theoretical considerations suggest that the risk of heparin-induced thrombocytopenia would be lower with low molecular weight heparins because it has fewer antigenic sites. There have been very few case reports of low molecular weight heparin-induced thrombocytopenia.[47,48] Warkentin and co-workers[28] measured the platelet counts and detected the presence of a heparin-induced thrombocytopenia IgG antibody in samples of patients enrolled in a randomized trial comparing unfractionated heparin with low molecular weight heparin for the prevention of venous thromboembolism after hip arthroplasty.[28] These investigators found a significantly lower incidence of both thrombocytopenia and the heparin-induced thrombocytopenia IgG antibody in patients who received low molecular weight heparin. The authors also reported higher odds of DVT in patients who developed heparin-induced thrombocytopenia.

Low molecular weight heparins have been proposed for the treatment of patients with heparin-induced thrombocytopenia who develop thrombotic complications.[49] The safety of this approach, however, is not entirely established in view of the high incidence of cross-reactivity between the low molecular weight heparins and the heparin-induced thrombocytopenia IgG antibody *in vitro*. Other alternatives in this situation are the use of lomoparan, a low molecular weight heparinoid, or ancrod, a defibrinating enzyme from the Malayan pit viper.

D. Osteoporosis

It has been suggested that low molecular weight heparins carry a lesser risk of osteoporosis than unfractionated heparin.[50] Unfortunately, the clinical evidence supporting this possibility is sparse and should be evaluated in properly designed studies.

VI. CLINICAL STUDIES

A. Prevention of Venous Thromboembolism

Low molecular weight heparins have been mainly evaluated in the prevention of venous thromboembolism in general surgical and orthopedic patients. Excellent meta-analyses and economic evaluations of these studies have been published (Table 6).[51-57] It is now established that venous thromboembolism prophylaxis in surgical patients reduces the incidence of DVT and death due to PE and its routine use has been advocated by five consensus conferences.[58-62]

1. General Surgery

Low doses of subcutaneous, unfractionated heparin is the traditional prophylactic method for patients above the age of 40 undergoing abdominopelvic surgery under general anesthesia for at least 30 minutes. Pooled analysis of these studies has shown a risk reduction for venous thromboembolism of approximately 65%.[34] The rates of DVT, PE and fatal PE with low dose heparin are low at 10%, 0.5% and 0.2%, respectively.

Several studies have compared low molecular weight heparins with placebo or unfractionated heparin in general surgical patients. Most studies have relied on ^{125}I-fibrinogen leg scanning for the assessment of DVT from approximately 10% with placebo to 3% with low molecular weight heparin.[51,52] This corresponds to a risk reduction of 70%.

Table 6
Meta-Analyses of Studies of Low Molecular Weight Heparin Prophylaxis versus Unfractionated Heparin with or without Dihydroergotamine in Surgical Patients.

Author	Surgical Group	Outcome	# Patients Studied		# Patients with Outcome (%)		Relative Risk (95% CI)
			LMWH	HEPARIN	LMWH	HEPARIN	
Nurmohamed 1992	General	DVT	3467	3411	184 (5.3)	230 (6.7)	0.79 (0.65-0.95)
		PE	2888	2843	9 (0.3)	20 (0.7)	0.44 (0.21-0.95)
		Bleeding*	1977	1966	52 (2.6)	51 (2.6)	1.01 (0.70)1.48)
	Orthopedic	DVT	672	622	93 (13.8)	132 (21)	0.68 (0.54-0.86)
		PE	590	582	10 (1.7)	24 (4.1)	0.43 (0.22-0.82)
		Bleeding	672	622	6 (0.9)	8 (1.3)	0.75 (0.26-2.14)
Jorgensen 1993	General	DVT	4425	4651	180 (4.1)	266 (5.7)	NM
		PE	4931	5186	8 (0.16)	31 (0.6)	0.13 (0.04-0.42)
	Orthopedic	DVT	1314	1272	222 (16.9)	275 (21.6)	0.67 (0.47-0.96)
		PE	1456	1408	4 (0.27)	19 (1.35)	NM
Leizorovicz 1992	General	DVT	5108	4575	248 (4.9)	267 (5.8)	0.86 (0.72-1.04)
		PE	4841	4305	12 (0.25)	25 (0.58)	0.62 (0.33-1.15)
		Bleeding	5108	4575	649 (12.7)	596 (13.0)	1.02 (0.90-1.16)

*Bleeding, major bleeding; LMWH, low molecular weight heparin; PE, pulmonary embolism.

There was a trend toward reduction of fatal PE with low molecular weight heparin. The incidence of fatal PE was 0.17% with placebo compared with 0.08% with low molecular weight heparin.[51] There was no difference in the incidence of major hemorrhage among the two treatment groups.[51] One study, however, reported a significantly higher incidence of wound hematomas with low molecular weight heparin.[63]

All comparative studies against unfractionated heparin entailed a once daily regimen of low molecular weight heparin versus low dose heparin, 5,000 U 12 hourly or 8 hourly. Some studies have compared combined modalities, i.e. low molecular weight heparin or low dose heparin plus elastic stockings or dihydroergotamine. Prophylaxis generally started 2 hours before surgery and was continued throughout the hospital stay. Pooled analysis of these studies show an overall lower incidence of DVT and PE with low molecular weight heparins. The clinical significance of these results, however, is debatable considering the very good results obtained with low dose heparin. On the other hand, the use of once daily regimen and a lesser risk of heparin induced thrombocytopenia are distinct advantages of low molecular weight heparins. Low molecular weight heparins may conceivably have a greater utility in more thrombogenic situations such as colorectal surgery or surgery for pelvic carcinoma but this needs to be studied further. Recent developments in the area of laparoscopic surgery may also change our approach to the prophylaxis of venous thromboembolism in general surgical patients in the future. Studies to evaluate the risk of venous thromboembolism after laparoscopic surgery are required.

No difference was observed in the incidence of major bleeding among the two treatment groups. However, a higher rate of bleeding or transfusion requirements associated with low molecular weight heparin use was observed in some studies as a result of the dosage regimen that was used.

2. Orthopedic Surgery

Major orthopedic surgery of the lower extremity became a logical field of investigation for the low molecular heparins in view of its highly thrombogenic and hemorrhagic potential. Low molecular weight heparins have been evaluated in hip arthroplasty, in knee arthroplasty and in patients with fractured hip.[51-54] Comparative studies have been performed versus placebo, unfractionated heparin or warfarin sodium. Studies that have compared low molecular weight heparins with placebo have reaffirmed the high incidence of DVT (i.e. 50%), without prophylaxis. Low molecular weight heparins achieved an overall risk reduction of approximately 50%. There was no difference in the incidence of major hemorrhage among the two treatment groups. Low molecular weight heparins were associated with an absolute rate of residual DVT of 20-25%, most of these involving the proximal veins.

Studies that have compared low molecular weight heparins with unfractionated heparin have used a variety of regimens. Unfractionated heparin regimens consisted of either 5,000 U BID-TID, the combination of heparin-dihydroergotamine, intermediate dose heparin (7,500 U BID) or adjusted dose heparin. Low molecular weight heparins were administered once or twice daily, with or without dihydroergotamine. Prophylaxis started either pre- or post-operatively, according to the study. Notwithstanding these variations in prophylaxis dosage regimens and schedule of administration, pooled analysis of these studies has shown an overall higher efficacy of low molecular weight heparins, with a risk reduction of approximately 20-25%. Of particular importance is the effect of low molecular weight heparins on the reduction of proximal DVT. Low molecular weight heparins reduce to approximately 5% the absolute rate of proximal DVT after hip arthroplasty.[54] No difference in major bleeding was observed between the two treatment groups.

Far fewer studies have been performed comparing low molecular weight heparins with oral anticoagulants. Hull and co-workers[64] compared a post-operative regimen of ILgiparin (75 U/kg subcutaneously once daily) with warfarin sodium (INR between 2.0 and 3.0) also commenced after surgery in patients undergoing hip or knee arthroplasty. The results showed a rate of DVT of 31% in the low molecular weight heparin group compared with 37% in the warfarin group. These results were statistically significant but their clinical significance is debatable. The incidence of major bleeding was 2.8% in the low molecular weight heparin group compared with 1.2% in the warfarin group. The results of this study must be interpreted in the context that a once daily regimen of low molecular weight heparin, started post-opertively, may be sub-optimal in orthopedic surgery. Additional studies are needed in this area.

B. Treatment of DVT

A number of studies have compared low molecular weight heparins with intravenous unfractionated heparin for the treatment of acute DVT of the lower extremity.[65-73] In all studies, intravenous heparin was adjusted according to the results of the aPTT and subcutaneous low molecular weight heparin was given once[72] or twice daily[65-71,73,74] at a fixed-dose regimen according to body weight. In all studies, except that by Hull, repeat venography was performed at the end of heparin treatment to assess the change in thrombus size. Four studies have documented prospectively the incidence of clinically relevant outcomes, i.e. death, major bleeding and recurrent venous thromboembolism.[69,70,72,73] The combined results of studies that have compared venography, pre- and post-heparin treatment, show a decrease in thrombus size in 65% of patients who received low molecular weight heparins compared with 50% for those treated with unfractionated heparin. The combined results of studies that have performed prospective follow-up, show a 2.7% incidence of recurrent venous thromboembolism in patients treated with low molecular weight heparins compared with 7% for those who received unfractionated heparin. Major hemorrhage occurred in approximately 1% of low molecular weight heparin-treated patients and in 3% of those who received unfractionated heparin. The finding of increased bleeding in the intravenous heparin group supports the results of animal studies discussed above and our overall understanding of the effect of low molecular weight heparins on hemostasis. It is possible that, in contrast to prophylaxis, we achieve the plasma levels of unfraction-unfractionated heparin required to cause increased bleeding whether it is via the inhibition of platelet function or any other mechanism. Mortality rate during follow-up was 4% in the low molecular weight heparin group compared with 8% in the unfractionated heparin group. All these long-term clinical outcomes are both clinically and statistically significant. The reason for this reduction in total mortality is not entirely clear at the present time. The results of these DVT treatment studies are very encouraging and open the avenue of treating this condition in the future on an outpatient basis. Further studies are needed in this area.

REFERENCES

1. **Beguin, S., Lindhout, T., Hemker, C.** The mode of action of heparin in plasma. *Thromb Haemost* 60, 457, 1988.
2. **Bigelow, W.** *Mysterious Heparin. The Key to Open Heart Surgery*. McGraw-Hill Ryerson, Scarborough, 1990, pp 205.
3. **Hirsh, J.** Heparin. *N Engl J Med* 324, 1565, 1991.
4. **Messmore, H., Griffin, B., Fareed, J., Coyne, E., Seghatchian, J.** In vitro studies of the interaction of heparin, low molecular weight heparin and heparinoids with platelets. *Ann NY Acad Sci* 556, 217, 1989.
5. **Bjornsson, T., Wolfram, K., Kitchell, B.** Heparin kinetics determined by three assay methods. *Clin Pharmacol Ther* 31, 104, 1982.
6. **Boneu, B., Dol, F., Caranobe, C., Sie, P., Houin, G.** Pharmacokinetics of heparin and related polysaccharides. *Ann*

NY Acad Sci 556, 282, 1989.

7. **Dawes, J., Bara, L., Billaud, E., Samama, M.** Relationship between biological activity and concentration of low-molecular weight heparin (PK10169) and unfractionated heparin after intravenous and subcutaneous administration. *Haemost* 16, 166, 1986.
8. **deSwart, C., Nijmeyer, B., Roelofs, J., Sixma, J.** Kinetics of intravenously administered heparin in normal humans. *Blood* 60, 1251, 1982.
9. **Duclos, J.** Proprietes biologiques de l'heparine. In: *L'Heparine.* Duclos, J. (ed), Masson, Paris, 1984, pp 1963.
10. **Hull, R., Raskob, G., Hirsh, J., Jay, R., Leclerc, J., Geerts, W., Rosenbloom, D., Sackett, D., Anderson, C., Harrison, L., Gent, M.** Continuous intravenous heparin compared with intermittent subcutaneous heparin in the initial treatment of proximal vein thrombosis. *N Engl J Med* 315, 1109, 1986.
11. **Glimelius, B., Busch, C., Hook, M.** Binding of heparin on the surface of cultured human endothelial cells. *Thromb Res* 12, 773, 1978.
12. **Laforest, M., Linhart-Colas, N., Vitaux-Guiraud, F., Bok, B., Samama, M., Marin, J., Imbault, F., Uzan, A.** Pharmacokinetics and biodistribution of technetium 99m labelled standard heparin and a low molecular weight heparin (enoxaparin) after intravenous injection in normal volunteers. *Br J Haematol* 77, 201, 1990.
13. **Sobel, M., McNeill, P., Carlson, P., Kermode, J., Adelman, B., Conroy, R., Marques, D.** Heparin inhibition of von Willebrand factor-dependent platelet function in vitro and in vivo. *J Clin Invest* 87, 1787, 1991.
14. **Lane, D., Denton, J., Flynn, A., Thunberg, L., Lindhal, U.** Anticoagulant activities of heparin oligosaccharides and their neutralization by platelet factor 4. *Biochem J* 218, 725, 1984.
15. **Lijnen, H., Hoylaerts, M., Collen, D.** Heparin binding properties of human histidine-rich glycoprotein. Mechanism and role in the neutralization of heparin in plasma. *J Biol Chem* 258, 3803, 1983.
16. **Preissner, K., Muller-Gerghaus, G.** Neutralization and binding of heparin by S-protein/vitronectin in the inhibition of factor Xa by antithrombin III. *J Biol Chem* 262, 1247, 1987.
17. **Young, E., Prins, M., Levine, M., Hirsh, J.** Heparin binding to plasma proteins, an important mechanism for heparin resistance. *Thromb Haemost* 67, 639, 1992.
18. **Chiu, H., Hirsh, J., Yung, W., Regoeczi, E., Gent, M.** Relationship between the anticoagulant and antithrombotic effects

of heparin in experimental venous thrombosis. *Blood* 49, 171, 1977.

19. **Heiden, D., Mileke, C., Rodvien, R.** Impairment by heparin of primary hemostasis and platelet {^{14}C} 5-hydroxytryptamine release. *Br J Haematol* 36, 427, 1977.
20. **Blajchman, M., Young, E., Ofosu, F.** Effects of unfractionated heparin, dermatan sulfate and low molecular weight heparin on vessel wall permeability in rabbits. *Ann NY Acad Sci* 556, 245, 1989.
21. **Fernandez, F., Nguyen, P., Van Ryn, J., Ofosu, F., Hirsh, J., Buchanan, M.** Hemorrhagic doses of heparin and other glycosaminoglycans induce a platelet defect. *Thromb Res* 43, 491, 1986.
22. **Turpie, A., Robinson, J., Doyle, D.** Comparison of high-dose with low-dose subcutaneous heparin to prevent left ventricular mural thrombosis in patients with acute transmural anterior myocardial infarction. *N Engl J Med* 320, 1989.
23. **Cruickshank, M., Levine, M., Hirsh, J., Roberts, R., Siguenza, M.** A standard heparin nomogram for the management of heparin therapy. *Arch Intern Med* 151, 333, 1991.
24. **Hull, R., Raskob, G., Rosenbloom, D., Lemaire, J., Pineo, G., Baylis, B.** Optimal therapuetic level of heparin therapy in patients with venous thromboembolism. *Arch Intern Med* 152, 1589, 1992.
25. **Raschke, R., Reilly, B., Guidry, J., Fontana, J., Srinivas, S.** The weight-based heparin nomogram compared with a "standard care" nomogram. *Ann Intern Med* 119, 874, 1993.
26. **King, D., Kelton, J.** Heparin-associated thrombocytopenia. *Ann Intern Med* 100, 535, 1984.
27. **Chang, J.** White clot syndrome associated with heparin-induced thrombocytopenia: A review of 23 cases. *Heart & Lung* 16, 403, 1987.
28. **Warkentin, T., Levine, M., Roberts, R., Gent, M., Horsewood, P., Kelton, J.** Heparin-induced thrombocytopenia is more common with unfractionated heparin than with low molecular weight heparin. *Thromb Haemost* 69, 911, 1993.
29. **Griffith, G., Nichols, G., Asher, J., Flanagan, B.** Heparin osteoporosis. *JAMA* 193, 85, 1965.
30. **DeSwiet, M.** Prolonged heparin therapy in pregnancy causes bone demineralisation. *Br J Obstet Gynaecol* 90, 1129, 1983.
31. **Raisz, L.** Local and systemic factors in the pathogenesis of osteoporosis. *N Engl J Med* 318, 818, 1988.
32. **Ginsberg, J., Kowalchuk, G., Hirsh, J.** Heparin effect on bone density. *Thromb Haemost* 64, 286, 1990.
33. **Dahlman, T., Lindvall, N., Hellgren, M.** Osteopenia in

pregnancy during long-term heparin treatment: a radiological study post-partum. *Br J Obstet Gynaecol* 97, 221, 1990.

34. **Collins, R., Scrimgeour, A., Yusuf, S., Peto, R.** Reduction in fatal pulmonary embolism and venous thrombosis by perioperative administration of subcutaneous heparin. *N Engl J Med* 1162, 1988.
35. **Andersson, L., Varrowcliffe, T., Holmer, E., Johnson, E., Sims, G.** Anticoagulant properties of heparin fractionated by affinity chromatography on matrix-bound antithrombin III and be gel filtration. *Thromb Res* 9, 575, 1976.
36. **Johnson, E., Kirkwood, T., Stirling, Y., Perez-Requejo, J., Ingram, G., Bangham, D., Brozovic, M.** Four heparin preparations: Anti-Xa potentiating effect of heparin after subcutaneous injection. *Thromb Haemost* 35, 586, 1976.
37. **Yin, E., Wessler, S., Stoll, P.** Biological properties of the naturally occurring antithrombotic and anticoagulant effect of low molecular weight heparins. *Thromb Res* 21, 169, 1981.
38. **Carter, C., Kelton, J., Hirsh, J., Cerskus, A., Santos, A., Gent, M.** The relationship between the hemorrhagic and antithrombotic properties of low molecular weight heparin in rabbits. *Blood* 59, 1239, 1982.
39. **Bendetowicz, A., Beguin, S., Caplain, H., Hemker, H.** Pharmacokinetics and pharmacodynamics of a low molecular weight heparin (enoxaparin) after subcutaneous injection, comparison with unfractionated heparin - A three way cross over study in human volunteers. *Thromb Haemost* 72, 305, 1994.
40. **Rosenberg, R.** Actions and interactions of antithrombin and heparin. *N Engl J Med* 292, 146, 1975.
41. **Colman, R., Scott, C., Pixley, R., De LaCadena, R.** Effect of heparin on the inhibition of the contact system enzymes. *Ann NY Acad Sci* 556, 95, 1989.
42. **Marciniak, E.** Factor Xa inactivation by antithrombin III: evidence for biological stabilization of factor Xa by factor V-phospholipid complex. *Br J Haematol* 24, 391, 1973.
43. **Frydman, A., Bara, L., LeRoux, Y., Woler, M., Chauliac, F., Samama, M.** The antithrombotic activity and pharmacokinetics of enoxaparine, a low molecular weight heparin, in humans given single subcutaneous doses of 20 to 80 mg. *J Clin Pharmacol* 28, 609, 1988.
44. **Hirsh, J., Levine, M.** Low molecular weight heparin. *Blood* 79, 1, 1992.
45. **Van Ryn-McKenna, J., Cai, L., Ofosu, F.A., Hirsh, J., Buchanan, M.R.** Neutralization of enoxaparine-induced bleeding by protamine sulfate. *Thromb Haemost* 63, 271, 1990.

46. **Salzman, E., Rosenberg, R., Smith, M., Lindon, J., Favreau, L.** Effect of heparin and heparin fractions on platelet aggregation. *J Clin Invest* 53, 563, 1980.
47. **Paille, F., Boccaccini, A., Korwin, J., Schmidt, C., Laprevote, M., Schmitt, J., Royer, R.** Thrombopenie sous heparine do bas poids moleculaire apres traitement par pentosane polysulfate. *Therapie* 43, 322, 1988.
48. **Eichinger, S., Kyrle, P., Brenner, B., Wagner, B., Kapiotis, S., Lechner, K., Kominger, H.** Thrombocytopenia associated with low-molecular weight heparin. *Lancet* 337, 1425, 1991.
49. **Leroy, J., Leclerc, M., Delahousse, B., Guerois, C., Foloppe, P., Gruel, Y., Toulemonde, F.** Treatment of heparin-associated thrombocytopenia and thrombosis with low molecular weight heparin (CY216). *Semin Thromb Haemost* 11, 326, 1985.
50. **Melissari, E., Parker, C., Wilson, N., Monte, G., Kanthou, C., Pemberton, K., Nicolaides, K., Barrett, J., Kakkar, V.** Use of low molecular weight heparin in pregnancy. *Thromb Haemost* 68, 652, 1992.
51. **Jorgensen, L., Will-Jorgensen, P., Hauch, O.** Prophylaxis of postoperative thromboembolism with low molecular weight heparins. *Br J Surg* 80, 689, 1993.
52. **Leizorovicz, A., Haugh, M., Chapuis, F., Samama, M., Boissel, J.** Low molecular weight heparin in prevention of perioperative thrombosis. *Br Med J* 305, 913, 1992.
53. **Nurmohamed, M., Rosendaal, F.S., Buller, H.R., Dekker, E., Hommes, D.W., Vandenbroucke, J.P.** Low molecular weight heparin versus standard heparin in general and orthopedic surgery: a meta-analysis. *Lancet* 340, 152, 1992.
54. **Mohr, D., Silverstein, M., Murtaigh, P., Harrison, J.** Prophylactic agents for venous thrombosis in elective hip surgery. *Arch Intern Med* 153, 2221, 1993.
55. **Menzin, J., Richner, R., Huse, D., Colditz, G., Oster, G.** Prevention of deep-vein thrombosis following total hip replacement surgery with enoxaparin versus unfractionated heparin: a pharmacoeconomic evaluation. *Ann Pharmacother* 28, 271, 1994.
56. **Anderson, D., O'Brien, B., Levine, M., Roberts, R., Wells, P., Hirsh, J.** Efficacy and cost of low-molecular weight heparin compared with standard heparin for the prevention of deep vein thrombosis after total hip arthroplasty. *Ann Intern Med* 119, 1105, 1993.
57. **O'Brien, B., Anderson, D., Goeree, R.** Cost-effectiveness of enoxaparin versus warfarin prophylaxis against deep vein

thrombosis after total hip replacement. *Can Med Assoc J* 150, 1083, 1992.

58. **Clagett, G., Saltzman, E., Wheeler, B., Anderson, F., Levine, M.** Prevention of venous thromboembolism. *Chest* 391S, 1992.
59. **Conference de Consensus.** Prophylaxie des thromboses veineuses profondes et des embolies pulmonaires postoperatoires. *Annales Francaises Anesthesie et Reanimation* 243, 1992.
60. **Nicolaides, A.N., Arcelus, J., Belcaro, G., Bergqvist, D., Borris, L.C., Buller, H.R., Caprini, J.A., Christopoulos, D., Clarke-Pearson, D., Clement, D., Colditz, G.A., Coleridge-Smith, P., Comerota, A.J., Cooke, E.D., Eklof, B., Fisher, C., Greenfield, L.J., Haas, S., Hull, R.D., Kakkar, V.V., Kalodiki, E., Lassen, M.R., Leclerc, J., Planes, A., Owen-Reece, A.R., Samama, M., Sasahara, A., Scurr, J.H., Ten Cate, G.W., Turpie, A.G., Widmer, L.** Prevention of venous thromboembolism. European Consensus Statement. *Int Angiol* 151, 1992.
61. **Lowe, G.D.O., Greer, I.A., Cooke, T.G., Dewar, E.P., Evans, M.J., Forbes, C.D., Mollan, R.A.B., Scurr, J.H., deSwiet, M.** Risk and prophylaxis for venous thromboembolism in hospital patients. Thromboembolic Risk Factors (THRIFT). *Br Med J* 567, 1992.
62. **Roberts, H.R., Adel, S., Bernstein, E.F., Buring, J., Demling, R.H., Fisher, L.D., Gonzales, O.A., Grover, J.W., Hanket, T.L., Hoaglund, F.T., Kaplan, K.L., Kitchens, C.S., Saltzman, H.A.** Prevention of venous thrombosis and pulmonary embolism. *JAMA* 747, 1986.
63. **Pezzuoli, G., Serneri, G., Settembrini, P., Coggi, G., Olivari, N., Buzzetti, G., Chierichetti, S., Scotti, A., Scatigna, M., Camovali, M.** Prophylaxis of fatal pulmonary embolism in general surgery using low-molecular weight heparin CY216: A multicentre, double-blind, randomized, controlled trial versus placebo (STEP). *Int Surg* 74, 205, 1989.
64. **Hull, R., Raskob, G., Pineo, G., Rosenbloom, D., Evans, W., Mallory, T., Anquist, K., Smith, F., Hughes, G., Green, D., Elliott, C., Panju, A., Brant, R.** A comparison of subcutaneous low-molecular weight heparin with warfarin sodium for prophylaxis against deep-vein thrombosis after hip or knee implantation. *N Engl J Med* 329, 1370, 1993.
65. **Bratt, G., Tornebohm, E., Granqvist, S., Aberg, W., Lockner, D.** A comparison between low molecular weight heparin Kabi2165 and standard heparin in the treatment of deep vein thrombosis. *Thromb Haemost* 85, 813, 1985.
66. **Faivre, R., Neuhart, E., Kieffer, Y., Toulemonde, F., Bassand, J., Maurat, J.** Subcutaneous administration of low molecular

weight heparin (CY222) compared with subcutaneous administration of standard heparin in patients with acute deep vein thrombosis. *Haemost* 58, 120, 1987 (Abstract).

67. **Bratt, G., Aberg, W., Johansson, M., Tornebohm, E., Granqvist, S., Lockner, D.** Two daily subcutaneous injections of Fragmin as compared with intravenous standard heparin in the treatment of deep vein thrombosis. *Thromb Haemost* 64, 506, 1990.
68. **Duroux, P., Ninet, J., Bachet, P.** A randomized trial of subcutaneous low molecular weight heparin (CY216) compared with intravenous heparin in the treatment of deep vein thrombosis. *Thromb Haemost* 65, 251, 1991.
69. **Prandoni, P., Lensing, A., Buller, H., Carta, M., Cogo, A., Vigo, M., Casara, D., Ruol, A.** Comparison of subcutaneous low-molecular weight heparin with intravenous standard heparin in proximal deep vein thrombosis. *Lancet* 339, 441, 1992.
70. **Lopaciuk, S., Meissner, A., Filipecki, S., Zamilska, K., Sowier, J., Cielielski, L., Bielawiec, M., Glowinski, S., Czestochowska, W.** Subcutaneous low molecular weight heparin versus subcutaneous unfractionated heparin in the treatment of deep vein thrombosis: a Polish multicentre trial. *Thromb Haemost* 68, 14, 1992.
71. **Hommes, D., Bura, A., Mazzolai, L., Buller, H., ten Cate, J.** Subcutaneous heparin compared with continuous intravenous heparin administration in the initial treatment of deep vein thrombosis. *Ann Intern Med* 116, 279, 1992.
72. **Hull, R., Raskob, G., Pineo, G., Green, D., Trowbridge, A., Elliott, C.** Subcutaneous low molecular weight heparin compared with continuous intravenous heparin in the treatment of proximal vein thrombosis. *N Engl J Med* 326, 975, 1992.
73. **Simonneau, G., Charbonnier, B., Decousus, H., Planchon, B., Ninet, J., Sie, P., Silsiguen, M., Combe, S.** Subcutaneous low-molecular weight heparin compared with continuous intravenous unfractionated heparin in the treatment of proximal deep vein thrombosis. *Arch Intern Med* 153, 1541, 1993.
74. **Holm, H., Ly, B., Handeland, G., Abildgaard, U., Arnesen, K., Gottschalk, P., Hoeg, V., Aandahl, M., Haugen, K., Laerum, F., Scheel, B., Sorland, O., Vinje, B.** Subcutaneous heparin treatment of deep venous thrombosis: A comparison on unfractionated and low molecular weight heparin. *Haemost* 16, 30, 1986.

Chapter 4

HEPARIN COFACTOR II AND THE PREVENTION AND TREATMENT OF THROMBOSIS

Michael R. Buchanan, Stephanie J. Brister and Frederick A. Ofosu

I. INTRODUCTION

Antithrombotic therapy, from the perspective of *anticoagulation,* currently involves the short-term administration of unfractionated heparin [or a low molecular weight heparin (LMWH) fraction], followed by a long-term course of an oral anticoagulant such as coumadin. Heparin or LMWH is given both to inhibit thrombin generation (prophylaxis) and/or to accelerate thrombin inhibition (treatment) by antithrombin III (ATIII). To maintain the efficacy of the heparin treatment, however, a long-term course of oral coumadin must be given to inhibit the synthesis of vitamin K-dependent procoagulant zymogens, thereby reducing the level of procoagulant substrates which will be available to contribute to thrombus formation. While such a therapeutic approach has provided widespread benefit for the prophylaxis and the treatment of thrombosis, there are a number of questions which remain unanswered. In particular, if heparin truly prevents additional thrombin generation and/or facilitates thrombin inhibition effectively, why is it necessary to provide long-term oral anticoagulation? Why do the patients remain at risk of recurrent thrombosis? Moreover, why do patients still suffer a thrombogenic event when on heparin therapy? Finally, why must patients be rendered hemostatically defective? i.e. hypocoagulated? It seems intuitively obvious that a course of "maximal" anticoagulant therapy at the time when diagnosis is confirmed should result in the correction of the underlying problem, thereby amelioriating thrombogenesis. Consequently, the patient should be able to return home with normal coagulation, i.e. neither being "hypercoagulated" nor "hypocoagulated", unless of course the patient has some genetically-related coagulopathy. This chapter will address these issues and assess the potential utility of thrombin inhibition by heparin cofactor II (HCII) and its catalysis by dermatan sulfate in treating established thrombosis.

II. WHY TARGET THROMBIN FOR INHIBITION?

The observations that heparin/ATIII reduces the risks of deep vein thrombosis[1], thrombus growth, acute closure of angioplasted coronary

0-8493-7649-1/95/$0.00+$.50

arteries[2] and facilitates reperfusion of occluded arteries during thrombolytic therapy[3], provide unrefutable evidence that thrombin is central to thrombogenesis, and that the accelerated inhibition of thrombin is critical for the prevention of thrombus formation and growth. It is also clearly evident that thrombin accelerates its own generation to further coagulation, and cleaves fibrinogen to initiate solid clot formation. Thrombin activates platelets, thereby facilitating platelet interactions with the injured vessel wall (see Chapter 1). Finally, thrombin acts as a potent mitogen[4], facilitating vessel wall hyperplasia and narrowing of the vessel wall. The feature which is common to both arterial and venous thrombosis is the formation of a solid thrombotic mass. Paramount to the formation of that solid thrombotic mass is the cleavage of fibrinogen to fibrin which, in turn, polymerizes into an insoluble mass. Thrombin is the only coagulant enzyme which directly clots fibrinogen, thereby forming a thrombus.[5] Considerable attention has been focused on surrogate markers of excessive coagulation such as elevated levels of Factor VII/VIIa, tissue factor expression, etc., suggesting that these markers represent and are directly responsible for the "prothrombotic" state.[6-8] There is no definitive evidence that the specific inhibition of any coagulant enzyme preceding thrombin in the coagulation system results in an effective inhibition of thrombin production to the level required to eliminate fibrin formation. For example, Ofosu et al.[9] demonstrated that the selective inhibition of Factor Xa by >80% has little, if any, effect on thrombin generation. Today, this result is not surprising since the existence of many positive feedback loops regulated by thrombin which enhances coagulation is now recognized (see Chapter 1). More importantly, however, Ofosu et al.[9] also demonstrated that almost complete inhibition of thrombin production could be achieved without any inhibition of Factor Xa (also see Chapter 1). Many investigators have shown that effective inhibition of thrombus formation can be achieved using thrombin inhibitors which have no effect on any other coagulant enzyme.[10-14] It seems logical, therefore, that the most direct approach to preventing thrombus formation is to regulate thrombin to minimize both its actions and its generation.

III. THE BASIS FOR ANTITHROMBOTIC THERAPY

Current anticoagulant therapy evolved from the observations that in the fluid phase, thrombin is inhibited predominantly by ATIII, and that heparin catalyzes this reaction (and to a lesser extent catalyzes the inhibition of other proteases by ATIII).[1] The ability of heparin to catalyze efficiently the inhibition of thrombin has been proposed to be the mechanism by which inhibition of thrombin-dependent amplification of the coagulation cascade is achieved (see Chapter 1). For example, heparin at less than 1 μg/ml inhibits the activation of prothrombin, inhibiting prothrombinase formation initiated by the addition of $CaCl_2$ to contact-activated plasma. Other anticoagulants, particularly heparin-related glycosaminoglycans, are also thought to achieve this effect. Heparan sulfate catalyzes thrombin/ATIII formation while dermatan sulfate catalyzes thrombin/HCII formation.[15] However, on a gravimetric basis, both of these compounds are less potent than heparin as catalysts of thrombin inhibition in circulating plasma. Consequently, heparin has become the anticoagulant of choice to the present day because of its ability to catalyze the rate of thrombin inhibition by ATIII by at least 1,000-fold.

While treatment of patients with heparin has undoubtedly been successful in saving lives and preventing morbid events associated with thrombus formation, heparin does not necessarily work in all patients in spite of efforts to optimize its use. Therefore, heparin may not be the ideal anticoagulant (see Chapters 5 and 6). This conclusion is based upon the observations that most patients requiring treatment for an initial thrombogenic event or for preventing the extension of an already formed thrombus, require not only short-term heparin treatment, but also long-term oral anticoagulation to prevent re-thrombosis.[1] Furthermore, 10-20% of patients who undergo major hip or knee replacement develop venous thrombosis, and 25-30% of coronary arteries in patients who undergo thrombolytic therapy or angioplasty reocclude despite the use of heparin/coumadin therapy.[16,17] These failures of heparin and its low molecular weight fractions in some of the above clinical settings appear to be related, in part, to the inability of heparin to inactivate effectively thrombin when bound to fibrin, platelets or an injured vessel wall surface.

IV. INHIBITION OF SURFACE-BOUND THROMBIN

A number of recent studies have increased our understanding of how heparin interacts with ATIII and thrombin under various conditions. As a consequence, these studies provide the rationale for replacing heparin with an alternate thrombin inhibitor. Specifically, the ability of heparin to catalyze thrombin inhibition by ATIII is impaired when thrombin binds to fibrin *in vitro*.[18,19] Similarly thrombin appears resistant to inhibition when thrombin binds to extracellular vascular components *in vitro*[20] or to freshly formed thrombi *in vivo*.[21] Fibrin-bound thrombin resistance to inhibition by heparin/ATIII appears to be related, in part, to overlapping binding sites on thrombin for heparin, ATIII and fibrin. Thus, in order for heparin to catalyze thrombin inhibition by ATIII, heparin must bind not only to ATIII at a high affinity site, but also to thrombin at an anionic exosite.[22] The thrombin exosite to which heparin binds, however, apparently overlaps the site to which thrombin binds fibrin, or becomes altered when thrombin binds fibrin. The exosite of thrombin for fibrin(ogen) is also important for the reaction of thrombin with ATIII. In contrast, fibrin-bound thrombin is not resistant to inhibition by HCII.[18-21]

V. THROMBIN HCII INHIBITION

A second endogenous inhibitor of thrombin in human plasma, namely, heparin cofactor II (HCII, Mr 65,600 dalton), inactivates thrombin but not other proteases of coagulation.[23] The normal concentration of HCII in the plasma is ≈1.2 ± 0.4 μmol/L or 80 ± 30 μg/mL. This concentration is ≈2-3 fold lower than the concentration of circulating ATIII ≈200 μg/ml. The half life of HCII, like ATIII, is ≈2 1/2 days.[24] When thrombin is added to or generated in plasma, either in the presence or absence of heparin, ≈90% of the thrombin is inhibited by ATIII and less than 10% is inhibited by HCII.[15] These observations give support to the concept that ATIII is by far a more important inhibitor of thrombin than HCII is.

HCII forms an equimolar complex with thrombin, but does not inhibit Factors VIIa, IXa, Xa, XIa, XIIa, kallikrein, activated protein C, plasmin, urokinase, tissue plasminogen activator, leukocyte elastase, gamma-subunit of nerve growth factor or epidermal growth factor binding protein.[25] HCII has been shown to inhibit α chymotrypsin, which recognizes the Leu-Ser reactive site peptide sequence of HCII.[26] [The HCII behavioural specificity contrasts markedly with the non-specific interactions of ATIII ± heparin. ATIII not only inhibits thrombin but also inhibits Factors Xa, IXa, XIIa, kallikrein].[27] Lysine residues appear to be essential for HCII activity.[26,28] Moreover, similar to the binding properties of heparin/ATIII/thrombin, heparin or dermatan sulfate must bind both to thrombin and to HCII for accelerated thrombin inhibition.[22,29,30] Finally, it should be noted that in the presence of dermatan sulfate, HCII catalyzes circulating thrombin >1,000-fold,[29] similar to extent of the catalytic effect of heparin on thrombin inhibition by ATIII. Until recently, little attention has been given to the potential antithrombotic effects associated with the catalytic inhibitory effects of HCII ± dermatan sulfate in the clinical setting. This may have been due, in part, to the observations that both in the absence or presence of glycosaminoglycans, thrombin in plasma is inhibited predominantly by ATIII. A number of recent studies now challenge that conclusion and suggest that in spite of their relatively weak anticoagulant activity *in vitro*, HCII-dependent anticoagulants have good antithrombotic properties with minimal hemorrhagic potential.

VI. INHIBITION OF THROMBIN BY HEPARIN COFACTOR II: EFFECT ON THROMBUS FORMATION/GROWTH IN THE EXPERIMENTAL SETTING

A. PREVENTION OF THROMBUS FORMATION

Historically, the recognition of the heterogeneity of heparin and the subsequent development of methods to produce LMWHs with high anti- Factor Xa to anti-thrombin ratios (see Chapter 3) resulted in a concerted effort to delineate the relative importance of the anti-thrombin and anti-Factor Xa activities of heparin fractions required to achieve an optimal antithrombotic effect. To that end, we performed studies to compare the relative effects of unfractionated heparin (which catalyzes thrombin and Factor Xa inhibition by ATIII), a low molecular weight heparin fraction (an octasaccharide which has only anti-Factor Xa activity) and dermatan sulfate (which only catalyzes thrombin inhibition by HCII, i.e. by a mechanism which was thought to be relatively ineffective).[10] The octasaccharide which only inhibits Factor Xa, was the least effective of the three as an antithrombotic agent. More importantly, dermatan sulfate (which not only has no anti-Factor Xa activity but also catalyzes thrombin inhibition by HCII) was at least as effective as heparin/ATIII as an antithrombotic.[10] These studies were not compatible with the then current dogma, namely, that inhibition of coagulant enzyme higher up the coagulation cascade is a more effective strategy to achieve an antithrombotic effect than inhibiting thrombin *per se*.[31] Subsequently, we examined the effectiveness of a variety of glycosaminoglycans. *Ex vivo* plasmas were obtained from animals injected with one of a number of glycosaminoglycans, including chondroitin-4-sulfate, chondroitin-6-sulfate, or a heparinoid. We found that regardless of the glycosaminoglycan tested, when given in a dose which caused a two-fold increase in thrombin inhibition *ex vivo*, all agents were equally effective in preventing the formation of experiment-induced thrombi in rabbits *in vivo*, irrespective of their anti-Factor Xa activities (or lack thereof).[32] These observations support the concept that the relative antithrombotic effect of any glycosaminoglycan can be determined by measuring its ability to catalyze thrombin inhibition *per se*, by ATIII alone, by HCII alone, or by both serpins. Glycosaminoglycan mixtures such as Sulodexide (a combination of fast moving heparin and dermatan sulfate, which catalyzes thrombin inhibition by ATIII and HCII simultaneously) have also been shown to have a synergistic effect on thrombin inhibition, thereby preventing thrombus formation when given in a dose lower than the dose of heparin or dermatan sulfate alone.[33,34] More importantly, when those agents which catalyze thrombin inhibition only by HCII are used, their antithrombotic effect is achieved with a dose which generates significantly less systemic anticoagulation, which, in turn, is associated with less bleeding side-effects.[35]

B. INHIBITION OF THROMBUS GROWTH

HCII-dependent inhibition of thrombin suppresses thrombus growth in rabbits more effectively than unfractionated heparin.[36-38] Dermatan sulfate inhibits prothrombin turnover (which is increased in rabbits with a pre-existing thrombus). Dermatan sulfate also inhibits thrombin accretion and fibrin deposition onto the thrombus more effectively than heparin.[19] Treating the rabbits with dermatan sulfate in a dose which induces minimal systemic anticoagulation (3 anti-thrombin units/kg) decreases prothrombin consumption, thrombin accretion and fibrin deposition on thrombi more effectively than unfractionated heparin, even when heparin is given in doses which generate 10 times greater systemic anticoagulation than dermatan sulfate. It should be noted that the specific thrombin inhibitor hirudin also has a comparable antithrombotic effect as dermatan sulfate, but only when given in a dose which generates a systemic anticoagulant effect comparable to heparin.[19] Since dermatan sulfate/HCII does not prevent thrombin generation *per se*[39], and its antithrombotic effect is achieved with minimal systemic anticoagulation, these results suggest that HCII/dermatan sulfate can effectively inactivate thrombin bound to fibrin and cell surfaces. These hypotheses have subsequently been validated by other investigators.[40,41] These results suggest that thrombin remains active when bound to a thrombus and accelerates further prothrombinase formation *in vivo*. Consequently, prothrombin turnover is markedly enhanced and additional fibrin formation is facilitated. These studies also provide the basis for the concept that inhibition of thrombin bound to a thrombus (or to an injured vessel wall) is fundamental for an irreversible antithrombotic effect. This concept would explain why heparin/ATIII, given as a short-term continuous course for the prevention of thrombus growth, requires further oral anticoagulant activity. It is likely that during the course of the heparin treatment, any thrombin generated by the pre-existing prothrombinase and remains within the circulation is effectively inhibited by heparin/ATIII. However, any thrombin which manages to bind to an injured vessel wall, traumatized tissue or a pre-existing thrombus escapes inhibition by heparin/ATIII.

C. ACUTE THROMBIN/HCII INHIBITION AND LONG-TERM EFFECTS ON VESSEL WALL HYPERPLASIA

The observation that thrombin bound to an injured vessel wall surface or fibrin monomer is resistant to inhibition by heparin/ATIII suggests that surface-bound thrombin can play a central role in maintaining continuous systemic hypercoagulation, thereby acting as a continuous stimulus at a specific site in the vasculature. The continuous presence of thrombin on the surface would enable the gradual formation of a solid thrombus not only by cleaving fibrinogen to fibrin, facilitating the laying down of a meshwork of fibrin fibres which could trap other blood components, but also by activating platelets which, in turn, recruit more blood cells to form the solid thrombus. Moreover, the thrombin could contribute to the release of mitogenic factors such as platelet derived growth factor by platelets at the site of vessel wall injury, or act directly as a mitogen[4], thereby facilitating chronic hyperplasia and subsequent vessel wall occlusion. Therefore, the utilization of a drug which would facilitate irreversible inhibition of surface-bound thrombin at the time of the vessel wall injury (or thrombus formation) should, in fact, ameliorate the long-term adverse effects of thrombin activity.

To test this possibility, we recently examined the effects of an acute treatment of dermatan sulfate or heparin, given acutely at the time of vessel wall injury, on thrombin inhibition and subsequent hyperplasia. Some rabbits were given the acute treatment of dermatan sulfate in a dose which generated minimal anticoagulation (≈0.2 U/ml of anti-thrombin activity, at the time of injury). Hyperplasia of injured carotid arteries measured 4 weeks later was reduced by 50%.[42] In contrast, when the animals were given an acute treatment of heparin in doses which generated ten-fold the anticoagulant activity at the time of injury, hyperplasia measured 4 weeks later was unaffected. These studies support the concept that effective thrombin inhibition at the time of injury can result in a long-term benefit without a long-term course of anticoagulation. To achieve this effect, however, it is necessary to catalyze HCII activity, not ATIII activity.

The inhibition of thrombin at the surface by HCII is also consistent with the biology of the vessel wall. Dermatan sulfate is a naturally occurring compound in the vessel wall.[43] It represents about 30% of the vascular glycosaminoglycans. HCII binds to dermatan sulfate associated with extracellular matrix components which are likely to be exposed following vessel wall injury.[44,45] Pretreatment of endothelial cells or smooth muscle cells with HCII prevents thrombin-induced cell pertubation. When ATIII + thrombin or HCII + thrombin are added to the media of endothelial or smooth muscle cells, thrombin-induced PGI_2 generation is inhibited in the presence of ATIII or HCII. However, if the cells are exposed first to ATIII and then washed, thrombin-induced PGI_2 generation is not inhibited. In contrast, if the cells are exposed to HCII and washed, thrombin-induced PGI_2 generation is inhibited. These results indicate that the HCII effect is associated with the binding of HCII to the cell surface. This inhibitory effect is enhanced in the presence of dermatan sulfate.[44]

D. THROMBOLYTIC SYNERGY WITH ATIII- AND HCII-DEPENDENT THROMBIN INHIBITORS

Thrombolytic agents such as tissue plasminogen activator (tPA) are used to restore patency of occluded coronary arteries in patients following acute myocardial infarction. Several clinical trials suggest that the rate of reperfusion with the thrombolytic therapy is enhanced in those patients who are given [tPA + heparin] as compared to those patients given tPA alone.[46-50] Heparin is thought to achieve this effect by preventing thrombus growth during the lytic treatment. If so, the enhanced effect of [tPA + heparin] should be achieved with lower doses of both tPA and heparin than those which are required to facilitate thrombolysis if either drug was given alone. An added benefit should also be associated with a reduced risk of bleeding with the combination [tPA + heparin] treatment.

However, early reocclusion develops in a significant number of patients despite the adjunct heparin treatment.[48] Furthermore, a long-term benefit of the adjunct treatment has not been well established since the frequency of reinfarction, recurrent ischemia and/or mortality do not appear to be reduced in those patients receiving the combination treatment as compared to tPA alone.[46,50-52] Finally, a number of clinical studies indicate that a high dose of heparin is necessary to enhance the tPA-induced thrombolysis.[48] Consequently, there are significant bleeding side-effects. The explanation for the differences in the expected and the observed results is not clearly understood.

The ability of tPA to accelerate plasminogen activation in the presence of fibrin *in vitro* has been reported to be impaired when heparin is added,[53,54] suggesting that tPA and heparin compete for similar sites on the fibrin-rich thrombus. However, other investigators suggest that tPA-induced fibrinolysis (measured *in vitro*) is not impaired when heparin is added.[55,56] Similar results are reported for studies *in vivo*. For example, Cercek et al.[57] found that a combination of [tPA + heparin] was more effective than tPA alone in reducing thrombus size in a canine model, but Haskel et al.[58] found that tPA-induced thrombolysis was not enhanced with adjunct heparin treatment (also in dogs). Agnelli et al.[59] found similar results in rabbits. Thus, neither *in vitro* nor *in vivo* experimental studies, nor prospective clinical studies have demonstrated unequivocally that tPA-induced thrombolysis is facilitated with adjunctive heparin.

The observation that thrombin bound to a thrombus or to a damaged vessel wall is resistant to inhibition by heparin/ATIII suggests a possible explanation of why higher than expected doses of heparin might be required to enhance tPA-induced thrombolysis. To determine if surface-bound thrombin may be involved in this process, we examined the relative benefits of heparin/ATIII and dermatan sulfate/HCII on tPA-induced lysis when each drug was given in doses which alone would have less than optimal antithrombotic effects.[60]

When rabbits with a pre-existing thrombus were infused with a dose of tPA which resulted in ≈40% lysis, adjunct heparin (30 U/kg/hr) did not enhance thrombolysis. In fact, when the heparin dose decreased to 10 U/kg/hr, tPA-induced thrombolysis was impaired, and the heparin dose had to be increased to 120 U/kg/hr to have any beneficial effect on thrombolysis (an increase 39 to 59%). While thrombolysis was increased, this effect was not due to a "synergistic effect". Moreover, bleeding was increased 20-fold.[60] In contrast, a low dose of dermatan sulfate (1.5 U/kg/hr), when given with the tPA infusion, increased thrombolysis by 50%.[60]

These observations demonstrate unequivocally that there is no synergism between "sub-optimal" doses of tPA and heparin, and are consistent with other *in vitro* and *in vivo* studies which demonstrate that the fibrinolytic effect of tPA is compromised in the presence of heparin. The observations that a low dose of dermatan sulfate does act synergistically with tPA while heparin does not, suggest that thrombin on the surface must be inhibited to prevent thrombus growth during thrombolysis.

These experimental studies are consistent with the clinical studies which demonstrate an enhanced benefit of tPA-induced thrombolysis with adjunct heparin therapy, because in those clinical studies 10,000 U of heparin was necessary to achieve increased thrombolysis, i.e. a dose greater than expected.[48] Not surprisingly, there was an increase in bleeding.[48] The observations that a lower dose of dermatan sulfate acts synergistically with tPA and this synergistic effect is achieved with minimal bleeding, suggest that inhibition of thrombin by HCII/dermatan sulfate is a safer approach to altering thrombolytic therapy.

VII. CONCLUSIONS

The observations of the unique protease specificity of HCII and its proteolytic effects in the absence or presence of dermatan sulfate compared to the non-specificity of heparin/ATIII,[25,27] suggest that HCII is, in fact, the more important inhibitor of thrombin which is compartmentalized in the extravascular space, or bound to the surfaces of injured blood vessel walls and a formed thrombus. It is becoming exquisitely clear that HCII inactivates thrombin on a surface much more effectively than ATIII.[18-21,34] The recent studies demonstrate that an acute treatment of dermatan sulfate/HCII effectively inhibits thrombin at the time of injury resulting in a chronic anti-hyperplasia effect[42], and suggest that HCII/thrombin inhibition may be the first order of thrombin regulation *in vivo*. Etiologically, this seems consistent since this effect can be achieved effectively at a local site of injury, without manifesting systemic anticoagulation. Moreover, the patient is not rendered hypocoagulable and at risk of bleeding. The lack of specificity of ATIII suggests that the ATIII/thrombin inhibition is a secondary phenomenon, associated perhaps with fail-safe mechanisms which keep in check a variety of activated procoagulants in the event that thrombin generation and its inhibition cannot be controlled locally at its site of initiation. Such an interpretation would also explain the potential utility of dermatan sulfate in a lower dose than heparin. It is interesting to note that agents which have the capacity to inhibit thrombin by ATIII and HCII simultaneously such as Sulodeexide can achieve an antithrombotic effect (either for thrombus prevention or thrombus growth) in doses which are substantially lower than the anticoagulant concentration which is required with heparin ATIII.[34]

VIII. FUTURE DIRECTIONS

If our interpretation of these recent experimental studies are correct, they have important implications in the clinical setting. Studies in Europe have demonstrated the efficacy of dermatan sulfate in preventing deep vein thrombosis following orthopedic hip surgery[61] or in preventing arterio-venous clot formation in patients undergoing hemodialysis.[62] Moreover, it is now recognized that plasma dermatan sulfate levels increase in normal pregnancy and decrease in patients with pre-eclampsia.[63] HCII activity, but not HCII antigenicity is decreased in insulin-dependent diabetic patients[64], i.e. in patients at an increased risk of thrombosis, although the clinical importance of this observation has yet to be clearly defined. HCII is also decreased in other settings in which the risk of thrombosis is increased.[65,66] Thus, the specificity of HCII inhibiting thrombin with site-specific activity, compared to a more global non-specificity of ATIII thrombin inhibition within the systemic circulation, gives credence to the concept that a better approach to achieving anticoagulant antithrombotic therapy is manipulating endogenous factors (HCII) to maintain "homeostasis", rather than employing agents with non-specific effects which are likely to inhibit thrombin throughout the entire system, thereby increasing the risk for bleeding. Obviously, thrombin is generated on a continuous basis in a normal, healthy individual to regulate homeostatic hemostasis. These individuals do not clot, presumably because coagulation is kept in check by the HCII/ATIII activity and do not bleed. Ideally, the best anticoagulant anti-thrombin would be that agent which will not render a patient hemostatically defective. Currently, most newer experimental approaches to anticoagulant therapy using agents such as argatroban, hirulog or other peptides which, while being as effective as dermatan sulfate in inhibiting surface-bound thrombin, may not achieve their anticoagulant effect without manifesting non-specific systemic effects.[67-69] Consequently, they have similar risks of bleeding as does heparin.[70] Only future clincal studies comparing the relative benefits of agents which work through the HCII pathway, with or without a synergism with the ATIII pathway, and direct thrombin inhibitors will determine which course of action achieves the best optimal antithrombotic effect in a variety of clinical settings.

REFERENCES

1. **Hirsh, J.** Heparin. *N Eng J Med* 324, 1565, 1991.
2. **Lincoff, A.M., Papma, J.J., Ellis, S.G., Hacker, J.A., Topol, E.J.** Abrupt vessel closure complicating coronary angioplasty: clinical, angiography and therapeutic profile. *J Am Coll Cardiol* 19, 926, 1992.
3. **Collen, D., Lijen, H.R.** Basic and clinical aspects of fibrinolysis and thrombolysis. *Blood* 78, 3114, 1991.
4. **Chen, L.B., Buchanan J.M.** Mitogenic activity of blood components/thrombin and prothrombin. *Proc Natl Acad Sci USA* 72, 131, 1975.
5. **Mann, K.G., Lorand, L.** Blood coagulation. *Methods Enzymol* 222, 1, 1993.
6. **Matsuda, M., Sugo, T., Sakata, Y., Murayama, H., Mimuro, J., Tanabe, S., Yoshitake, S.A.** Thrombotic state due to an abnormal protein C. *N Engl J Med* 319, 1265, 1988.
7. **Demers, C., Ginsberg, J., Henderson, P., Ofosu, F.A., Weitz, J., Blajchman, M.** Measurement of markers of activated coagulation in antithrombin III deficient subjects. Thromb Haemost 67, 542, 1992.
8. **Amelsberg, A., Zurborn, K.H., Gartner, U., Kiehne, K.H., Preube, A-K., Bruhn, H.D.** Influence of heparin treatment on biochemical markers of an activation of the coagulation system. Thromb Res 66, 121, 1992.
9. **Ofosu, F.A., Blajchman, M.A., Modi, G.J., Smith, L.M., Buchanan, M.R., Hirsh, J.** The importance of thrombin inhibition for the expression of the anticoagulant activities of heparin, dermatan sulphate, low molecular weight heparin and pentosan

polysulphate. *Br J Haematol* 60, 695, 1985.

10. **Buchanan, M.R., Boneu, B., Ofosu, F., Hirsh, J.** The relative importance of thrombin inhibition and Factor Xa inhibition to the antithrombotic effects of heparin. *Blood* 65, 198, 1985.
11. **Brill-Edwards, P., Van Ryn-McKenna, J., Cai, L., Ofosu, F., Buchanan, M.R.** Prevention of thrombus growth by antithrombin III-dependent and two direct thrombin inhibitors in rabbits: Implications for antithrombotic therapy. *Thromb Haemost* 68, 424, 1992.
12. **Van Ryn-McKenna, J., Merk, H., Muller, T.H., Buchanan, M.R., Eisert, W.G.** The effects of heparin and annexin V on fibrin accretion after injury in the jugular veins of rabbits. *Thromb Haemost* 69, 227, 1993.
13. **Bacher, P., Walenga, J.M., Iqbal, O., Bajusz, S., Breddin, K., Fareed, J.** The antithrombotic and anticoagulant effects of a synthetic tripeptide and recombinant hirudin in various animal models. *Thromb Res* 71, 251, 1993.
14. **Maraganore, J.M., Chao, B., Joseph, M.L., Jablonski, J., Ramachandran, K.L.** Anticoagulant activity of synthetic hirudin peptides. *J Biol Chem* 264, 8692, 1989.
15. **Ofosu, F.A., Fernandez, F., Buchanan, M.R., Petitou, M., Boneu, B.** Respective role of antithrombin III and heparin cofactor II in the *in vitro* anticoagulant effect of heparin and of various sulphated polysaccharides. *Br J Haematol* 64, 707, 1986.
16. **Hirsh, J., Levine M.** Prevention of venous thrombosis in patients undergoing major orthopedic surgical procedures. *Br J Clin Pract* 65, 2, 1989.
17. **LeFeuvre, C., Bonan, R., Cote, G., Crepeau, J., DeGuise, P., Lesperance, J., Theroux, P.** Five- to ten-year outcome multivessel percutaneous transluminal coronary angioplasty. *Am J Cardiol* 71, 1153, 1993.
18. **Hogg, P.J., Jackson, C.M.** Fibrin monomer protects thrombin from inactivation by heparin-antithrombin III: Implications for heparin efficacy. *Proc Natl Acad Sci USA* 86, 3619, 1989.
19. **Okwusidi, J.I., Anvari, N., Kulczycky, M., Blajchman, M.A., Buchanan, M.R., Ofosu, F.A.** Fibrin moderates the catalytic action of heparin but not that of dermatan sulfate on thrombin inhibition in human plasma. *J Lab Clin Med* 117, 359, 1991.
20. **Bar-Shavit, R., Eldor, A., Vlodavsky, I.** Binding of thrombin to subendothelial extracellular matrix. *J Clin Invest* 1989, 1096, 1989.
21. **Okwusidi, J., Falcone, M., Van Ryn-McKenna, J., Hirsh, J., Ofosu, F.A., Buchanan, M.R.** *In vivo* catalysis of thrombin inhibition by antithrombin III or heparin cofactor II and anti-

thrombotic effect: differential effects of unfractionated heparin and dermatan sulphate. *Thromb Haemorrh Dis* 1/2, 77, 1990.
22. **Griffith, M.J.** Heparin-catalyzed inhibitor/protease reactions: kinetics evidence for a common mechanism of action of heparin. *Proc Natl Acad Sci USA* 80, 5460, 1983.
23. **Tollefsen, D.M., Blank, M.K.** Detection of a new heparin-dependent inhibitor of thrombin in human plasma. *J Clin Invest* 68, 689, 1981.
24. **Dupouy, P.S.D., Pichon, J., Boneu, B.** Turnover study of heparin cofactor II in healthy man. *Thromb Haemost* 54, 635, 1985.
25. **Parker, K.A., Tollefsen, D.M.** The protease specificity of heparin cofactor II. *J Biol Chem* 260, 3501, 1985.
26. **Church, F.C., Noyes, C.M., Griffith, M.J.** Inhibition of chymotrypsin by heparin cofactor II. *Proc Natl Acad Sci USA* 82, 6431, 1985.
27. **Dupouy, P.S.D., Pichon, J., Boneu, B.** Turnover study of heparin cofactor II in healthy man. *Thromb Haemost* 54, 635, 1985.
28. **Church, F.C., Griffith M.J.** Evidence for essential lysines in heparin cofactor II. *Biochem Biophys Res Comm* 124, 745, 1984.
29. **Tollefsen, D.M., Pestka, C.A., Monafo, W.J.** Activation of heparin cofactor II by dermatan sulfate. *J Biol Chem* 258, 6713, 1983.
30. **Lindahl, U., Hook, M.** Glycosaminoglycan and their binding to biological macro molecules. *Annu Rev Biochem* 47, 385, 1978.
31. **Hirsh, J., Ofosu, F.A., Buchanan, M.R.** Rationale behind the development of low molecular weight heparin derivatives. *Semin Thromb Hemost* 11, 13, 1985.
32. **Fernandez, F.A., Buchanan, M.R., Hirsh, J., Fenton, J.W., II, Ofosu, F.A.** Catalysis of thrombin inhibition provides an index for estimating the antithrombotic potential of glycosaminoglycans in rabbits. *Thromb Haemost* 57, 286, 1987.
33. **Buchanan, M.R., Brister, S.J., Ofosu, F.A.** Prevention and treatment of thrombosis. Novel strategies arising from our understanding the healthy endothelium. *Wien Klin Wochenschr* 105, 309, 1993.
34. **Buchanan, M.R., Liao, P., Smith, L.J., Ofosu, F.A.** Prevention of thrombus formation and growth by antithrombin III and heparin cofactor II-dependent thrombin inhibitors: importance of the heparin cofactor II. *Thromb Res* 74, 463, 1994.
35. **Van Ryn-McKenna, J., Ofosu, F.A., Hirsh, J., Buchanan, M.R.** Antithrombotic and bleeding effects of glycosaminoglycans with different degrees of sulphation. *Br J Haematol* 71, 265, 1989.

36. **Van Ryn-McKenna, J., Ofosu, F.A., Gray, E., Hirsh, J., Buchanan, M.R.** Effects of dermatan sulfate and heparin on inhibition of thrombus growth *in vivo*. *Ann NY Acad Sci* 556, 304, 1989.
37. **Ofosu, F.A., Fernandez, F., Gauthier, D., Buchanan, M.R.** Heparin cofactor II and other endogenous factors in the mediation of the antithrombotic and anticoagulant effects of heparin and dermatan sulfate. *Semin Thromb Hemost* 11, 133, 1985.
38. **Gray, E., Cesmeli, S., Lormeau, J.C., Davies, A.B., Lane, D.A.** Low affinity heparin is an antithrombotic agent. *Thromb Haemost* 71, 203, 1994.
39. **Ofosu, F.A., Buchanan, M.R., Anvari, N., Smith, L.M., Blajchman, M.A.** Plasma anticoagulant mechanisms of heparin, heparan sulfate, and dermatan sulfate. *Ann NY Acad Sci* 556, 123, 1989.
40. **Bendayan, P., Boneu, B., Boccalon, H.** Dermatan sulfate is a more potent inhibitor of clot bound thrombin than unfractionated and low molecular weight heparins. *Thromb Haemost* 69, 656, 1993.
41. **Cadroy, Y., Dol, F., Caranobe, C., Petitou, M., Lormeau, J.C., Sie, P., Choay, J., Boneu, B.** Standard heparin enhances the antithrombotic activity of dermatan sulfate in the rabbit but CY216 does not. *Thromb Haemost* 59, 295, 1988.
42. **Buchanan, M.R., Brister, S.J., Laio, P., Warnke, C., Ofosu, F.A.** Effects of heparin and dermatan sulfate on injured vessel wall hyperplasia and vessel wall occlusion. *Thromb Haemost* 69, 950, 1993.
43. **Muratak,** Distribution of acidic glycosaminoglycans, lipids and water in normal human cerebral arteries of various ages. *Stroke* 16, 685, 1985.
44. **Hayashi, T., Kaji, T., Hayakawa, Y., Niiya, K., Sakamoto, M., Sakuragawa, N.** Inhibitory effect of heparin cofactor II on thrombin-stimulated prostacyclin production by cultured vascular smooth muscle cells. *Thromb Res* 64, 321, 1991.
45. **Kaji, T., Itah, F., Hayakawa, Y., Oguma, Y., Sakuragawa, N.** Interaction of thrombin with heparin cofactor II and antithrombin III on prostacyclin production by cultured endothelial cells. *Thromb Res* 56, 99, 1989.
46. **Topol, E.J., George, B.S., Kerelakee, D.J.** A randomized controlled trial of intravenous tissue plasminogen activator and early intravenous heparin in acute myocardial infarction. *Circ* 79, 281, 1989.

47. **TIMI Study Group.** Comparison of invasive and conservative strategies after treatment with intravenous tissue plasminogen activator in acute myocardial infarction. Results of thrombolysis in acute myocardial infarction (TIMI) phase II trial. *N Engl J Med* 320, 618, 1989.
48. **Prins, M.H., Hirsh, J.** Heparin as an adjunctive treatment after thrombolytic therapy for acute myocardial infarction. *Am J Cardiol* 67, 3A, 1991.
49. **Schaer, D.H., Ross, A.M., Wasserman, A.G.** Reinfarction, recurrent angina and reocclusion after thrombolytic therapy. *Circ* 76, 1157, 1987.
50. **Bleich, S.D., Nichols, T.C., Schumacher, R.R., Cooke, D.H., Tate, D.A., Teichman, S.L.** Effect of heparin on coronary arterial patency after thrombolysis with tissue plasminogen activator in acute myocardial infarction. *Am J Cardiol* 66, 1412, 1990.
51. **Hsia, J., Hamilton, W.P., Kleiman, N., Roberts, R., Chaitman, B.R., Ross, A.M.** A comparison between heparin and low-dose aspirin and adjunctive therapy with tissue plasminogen activator for acute myocardial infarction. *N. Engl J Med* 323, 1433, 1990.
52. **GISSI-2 (Gruppo Italiano per lo Studio Della Sopravvivenza Nell'Infarto Miocardio).** In-hospital mortality and clinical course of 20,891 patients with suspected acute myocardial infarction randomized between alteplase and streptokinase with or without heparin. *Lancet* 336, 71, 1990.
53. **Andrade-Gordon, P., Strickland, S.** Interaction of heparin with plasminogen activators and plasminogen: Effects on the activation of plasminogen. *Biochemistry* 25, 4033, 1986.
54. **Pacques, E.P., Stohr, H.A., Heimburger, N.** Study on the mechanism of action of heparin and related substances on the fibrinolytic system: Relationship between plasminogen activators and heparin. *Thromb Res* 42, 797, 1986.
55. **Fry, E.T.A., Sobel, B.E.** Lack of interference by heparin with thrombolysis or binding of tissue type plasminogen activator to thrombi. *Blood* 71, 1346, 1988.
56. **Weitz, J.I., Kuint, J., Leslie, B., Hirsh, J.** Standard and low molecular weight heparin have no effect on tissue plasminogen activator induced plasma clot lysis or fibrinogenolysis. *Thromb Haemost* 65, 541, 1991.
57. **Cercek, B., Lew, A.S., Hod, H., Yano, J., Reddy, N., Ganz, W.** Enhancement of thrombolysis with tissue type plasminogen activator by pretreatment with heparin. *Circ* 74, 583, 1988.
58. **Haskel, E.J., Rragner, N.A., Sobel, B.E., Abenahein, D.R.** Relative efficacy of anti-thrombin compared with antiplatelet agents in accelerating coronary thrombolysis and preventing

early reocclusion. *Circ* 83, 1048, 1991.

59. **Agnelli, G., Pascucci, C., Cosmi, B., Nenol, G.** Effects of therapeutic doses of heparin on thrombolysis with tissue type plasminogen activator in rabbits. *Blood* 76, 2030, 1990.
60. **Van Ryn-McKenna, J., Ofosu, F.A., Buchanan, M.R.** The effects of heparin and dermatan sulphate on tPA-induced thrombolysis and blood loss in rabbits. *Fibrinolysis* 7, 75, 1993.
61. **Agnelli, G., Cosmi, B., DiFilippo, P., Ranucci, V., Veschi, F., Longetti, M., Renga, C., Barzi, F., Gianese, F.A., Lupattelli, L., Rinonapoli, E., Nenci, G.G.** A randomised, double-blind, placebo-controlled trial of dermatan sulphate for prevention of deep vein thrombosis in hip fracture. *Thromb Haemost* 67, 203, 1992.
62. **Ryan, K.E., Lane, D.A., Flynn, A., Ireland, H., Boisclair, M., Sheppard, J., Curtis, J.R.** Antithrombotic properties of dermatan sulphate (MF701) in haemodialysis for chronic renal failure. *Thromb Haemost* 68, 563, 1992.
63. **Andrew, M., Mitchell, L., Paes, B., Berry, L., Burrows, R., Khambalia, B., Ofosu, F.A.** An anticoagulant dermatan sulphate proteoglycan circulates in the pregnant woman and her fetus. *J Clin Invest* 89, 321, 1992.
64. **Ceriello, A., Quatraro, A., Russo, P.D., Marchi, E., Milani, M.R., Giugliano, D.** Evidence for a reduced heparin cofactor II biological activity in diabetes. *Haemost* 20, 357, 1990.
65. **Matsuo, T., Kazuomi, K., Sakamoto, S., Yamada, T., Miki, T., Hirase, T., Kobayashi, H.** Hereditary heparin cofactor II deficiency and coronary artery disease. *Thromb Res* 65, 495, 1992.
66. **Tollefsen, D.M., Pestka, C.A.** Heparin cofactor II activity in patients with disseminated intravascular coagulation and hepatic failure. *Blood* 66, 769, 1985.
67. **Yamashita, T., Yamamoto, J., Sasaki, Y., Matsuoka, A.** The antithrombotic effect of low molecular weight synthetic thrombin inhibitors, argatroban and PPACK, on he-ne laser-induced thrombosis in rat mesenteric microvessels. *Thromb Res* 69, 93, 1993.
68. **Jang, I.K., Gold, H.K., Leinbach, R.C., Fallon, J.T., Collen, D.** In vivo thrombin inhibition enhances and sustains arterial recanalization with recombinant tissue type plasminogen activator. *Circ Res* 67, 1552, 1990.
69. **Agnelli, G., Buchanan, M.R., Fernandez, F., Van Ryn, J., Hirsh, J.** Sustained thrombolysis with DNA-recombinant tissue type plasminogen activator in rabbits. *Blood* 66, 339, 1985.

70. **Carter, C.J., Kelton, J.G., Hirsh, J., Fenton, J.W., II, Ofosu, F.A., Gent, M.** The relationship between hemorrhagic and antithrombotic properties of low molecular weight heparin in rabbits. *Blood* 59, 1239, 1982.

Chapter 5

DEVELOPMENT AND RATIONALE FOR THE USE OF DIRECT THROMBIN INHIBITORS IN THE PREVENTION AND TREATMENT OF ARTERIAL AND VENOUS THROMBOSIS

Jeffrey S. Ginsberg

I. INTRODUCTION

Thrombosis is a leading cause of mortality in Western societies. Several advances in antithrombotic therapy have been made in recent years, including optimizing the use of unfractionated heparin, several low molecular weight heparins, heparinoids, and warfarin to prevent and treat thromboembolism.[1] Nonetheless, the use of these agents is associated with a significant risk of bleeding.[1,2] Furthermore, for patients with deep venous thrombosis (DVT), long-term warfarin therapy is required, following cessation of unfractionated or low molecular weight heparin therapy, to prevent recurrence of DVT.[1] Finally, 15-25% of patients who have major hip or knee surgery develop DVT[3], and up to 30% of coronary arteries of patients who undergo thrombolytic therapy or 5-10% of coronary arteries of patients who undergo angioplasty reocclude, despite the use of unfractionated or low molecular weight heparin.[4,5] These observations indicate that while unfractionated and low molecular weight heparins can effectively prevent thrombus formation and growth, they are not ideal. It is likely that rethrombosis following cessation of heparin-like compounds is related to their inability to inhibit clot-bound thrombin completely, or their inability to inactivate prothrombinase, both of which can be the stimuli for the thrombotic event and subsequent reocclusion.[6]

Recent studies provide some explanations for the ineffectiveness of heparin and suggest alternative approaches.[6-8] When thrombin is bound to fibrin or to injured vessel wall surfaces, it becomes resistant to inhibition by heparin/antithrombin III, but remains relatively more susceptible to inactivation by direct thrombin inhibitors, such as hirudin and hirulog.[6-8] The thrombin bound to fibrin produces more fibrin in two ways: direct proteolysis, and perhaps more importantly by activating Factor XI, Factor V, and Factor VIII to facilitate prothrombinase formation.[9] Heparin is effective clinically because it catalyzes the inhibition of thrombin to inhibit these positive amplification loops of coagulation before it becomes entrapped by fibrin or platelets. However, because heparin cannot inhibit fibrin-bound thrombin as effectively as it can inhibit free thrombin, once heparin is discontinued, the enzymatically competent fibrin-bound

0-8493-7649-1/95/$0.00+$.50

thrombin can activate Factors V and VIII. This enhances prothrombinase formation, thereby facilitating thrombus growth and extension.

Experimental studies have demonstrated that effective inhibition of both thrombus formation and growth can be achieved using agents which inactivate thrombin directly, e.g. hirudin and hirulog. Hirudin and hirulog appear to access and inactivate clot-bound thrombin more effectively than heparin.[6,8]

Direct thrombin inhibitors are molecules that inactivate thrombin by forming 1:1 stoichiometric complexes with thrombin. For the purposes of this chapter, the term "direct thrombin inhibitor" will be used to refer only to exogenous direct thrombin inhibitors, such as hirudin and its fragments, and not to endogenous direct thrombin inhibitors, such as antithrombin III and heparin cofactor II. In addition, only hirudin and hirulog, a derivatized carboxyl terminal fragment of hirudin, will be reviewed since to date the only large clinical trials which have been published have used these agents. Clinical evaluation of other direct thrombin inhibitors, some of which may prove to be superior to hirudin and hirulog, is still ongoing.

Promising results with direct thrombin inhibitors in experimental animals have encouraged the development of these and other direct anti-thrombins for clinical use in order to address three main clinical questions: 1) Do direct thrombin inhibitors have advantages over unfractionated and low molecular weight heparin and warfarin therapy in patients with venous thrombosis? 2) Are direct thrombin inhibitors given to patients undergoing major orthopedic surgery to reduce the incidence of DVT to less than 15-25% (the rates obtained with warfarin and low molecular weight heparins) safe? 3) Are these agents more beneficial clinically in patients with symptomatic coronary artery disease when given specifically to prevent reocclusion in patients undergoing angioplasty, in patients with unstable angina or in patients receiving thrombolytic therapy for a myocardial infarction?

II. CLINICAL STUDIES OF DIRECT THROMBIN INHIBITORS

Although several direct thrombin inhibitors have been developed or are in various phases of clinical development, as of January 1994, the only large published clinical studies are those in which either hirulog or hirudin was used. Hirulog is a bivalent 20 amino acid synthetic peptide inhibitor of thrombin which is a modified carboxyl tail of hirudin. The results of several Phase 2 clinical trials of hirulog and hirudin have been published and several large studies are ongoing. These agents have been used for the treatment of patients with venous thrombosis or unstable angina, and for the prevention of reocclusion of the coronary arteries after angioplasty or thrombolytic therapy.

A. PREVENTION OF VENOUS THROMBOSIS AFTER ORTHOPEDIC SURGERY

It is likely that small thrombi form intra-operatively in many patients undergoing major orthopedic surgery. Thrombus growth is probably triggered by cell-bound prothrombinase and thrombin bound to fibrin which remains enzymatically active.[6] Clot-bound thrombin is resistant to inactivation by heparin-antithrombin III, an observation which may explain why heparin-related compounds are limited in their ability to prevent DVT in patients undergoing major orthopedic surgery.[6] Heparin does not catalyze the inactivation of Factor Xa at a rate which inhibits prothrombin activation once the enzyme becomes incorporated into prothrombinase.[10] In contrast to heparin, antithrombin III-independent thrombin inhibitors can readily inactivate clot-bound thrombin, thereby raising the possibility that these agents may be better than heparin and low molecular weight heparins at preventing DVT in high risk patients.[6,8] While the direct thrombin inhibitors are unlikely to inactivate pre-formed prothrombinase, they will, like heparin, inhibit the formation of new prothrombinase.

Two clinical trials of direct thrombin inhibitors for the prevention of venous thrombosis after major hip and/or knee surgery, one with hirulog and one with hirudin, have been published. The first study was a Phase 2 dose-ranging study in patients undergoing major elective knee or hip surgery or surgery for hip fracture.[11] Hirulog was started post-operatively and was given subcutaneously for up to 14 days. All patients underwent mandatory bilateral venography prior to discharge to determine the presence or absence of DVT.

The study enrolled 222 patients; 177 (79.7%) had technically adequate bilateral venography (176 patients) or pulmonary embolism without venography (1 patient) and were included in the primary analysis of efficacy. The rates of venous thromboembolism observed with each of the hirulog regimens are listed in Table 1. The overall DVT rates seen in the first 4 regimens were high, but fell substantially in the last regimen. The difference in overall DVT rates between the first 4 regimens (43%) and the last regimen (17%) is highly significant ($p = 0.004$). As with the overall DVT rates, the difference in proximal DVT rates between the first 4 regimens (20%) and the last regimen (2%) of hirulog is highly significant ($p = 0.002$). Two patients suffered non-fatal pulmonary embolism during the study; both had received hirulog 0.6 mg/kg twice daily.

Only 3 patients (1.4%) suffered major bleeding events; 1 patient received hirulog 0.6 mg/kg q12/hour, the second received hirulog 1.0

Table 1
DVT Rates in a Phase 2 Study of Hirulog in Patients Undergoing Major Hip or Knee Surgery

Dose Regimen of Hirulog

DVT Rate	0.3mg/kg q12h (n=17)	0.6mg/kg* q12h (n=54)	1.0/0.6mg/kg q12h** (n=40)	1.0mg/kg q12h (n=20)	1.0mg/kg q8h (n=46)
Overall	10 (59%)	23 (43%)	16 (40%)	7 (35%)	8 (17%)
Proximal	7 (41%)	9 (17%)	6 (15%)	4 (20%)	1 (2%)

*Includes 2 patients who had pulmonary embolism; 1 who had proximal DVT by venography and 1 who did not undergo venography. The latter was considered positive for both overall and proximal DVT. **1.0 mg/kg q12 hour x 3 day, followed by 0.6 mg/kg for up to 11 days.

mg/kg q12/hour for 3 days followed 0.6 mg/kg q12/hour, and the third received hirulog 1.0 mg/kg q8/hour. Three patients suffered minor bleeding events; two patients who had received hirulog 0.6 mg/kg q12/hour and one received 1.0 mg/kg q12/hour.

The activated partial thromboplastin time (aPTT) results, measured 2 hours following hirulog administration, are provided in Table 2. In addition, the regimen involving 8 hourly injections of hirulog produced an anticoagulant effect throughout the day in most patients whereas 12 hourly injections did not. The presence of a weak anti-hirulog response was demonstrated in only 2 patients (1.1%) who had no adverse clinical or laboratory findings associated with these responses.

Two points are noteworthy in this study. First, the only dose of hirulog which was effective prolonged the aPTT at all times in between injections, suggesting that there must be significant circulating plasma levels of the hirulog at all times in order for the drug to be effective clinically. The second novel observation also pertains to the aPTT results. The effective dose of hirulog produced substantial and consistent prolongation of the aPTT. Sustained anticoagulation is not required to achieve clinical efficacy with heparin when heparin is used prophylactically. Thus, there is evidence from other studies that if heparin had been used in a dose which prolonged the aPTT to the same extent as the hirulog, the heparin treatment would have resulted in considerably more bleeding than that seen with hirulog.[12] The low incidence of bleeding associated with hirulog administration is encouraging and suggests that potential improvements in clinical

Table 2
aPTT Results on Day 2* in a Phase 2 Study of Hirulog in Patients Undergoing Major Hip or Knee Surgery

	Dose Regimen of Hirulog				
	0.3mg/kg q12h (n=18)	0.6mg/kg q12h (n=68)	1.0/0.6mg/kg q12h** (n=49)	1.0mg/kg q12h (n=28)	1.0mg/kg q8h (n=59)
aPTT (secs)					
Mean	41.5	46.5	54.6	51.4	49.1
S.D.	14.2	10.7	10.6	14.7	12.1

* Performed on plasma samples taken 2 hours after the morning dose of hirulog; control value = 32-34 seconds. ** 1.0 mg/kg q12 hour x 3 day, followed by 0.6 mg/kg for up to 11 days.

efficacy may not come at the expense of an increased risk of bleeding. These findings suggest that the effect of different antithrombotic agents cannot be standardized on the basis of a comparison of the aPTT with heparin therapy.

In the second dose-ranging study, recombinant hirudin, started preoperatively, was administered twice daily to 48 patients undergoing elective total hip replacement.[13] Twelve patients received 10 mg of hirudin twice daily, 12 received 15 mg twice daily, 21 received 20 mg twice daily, and 3 received 40 mg twice daily. Two of the 3 patients receiving the highest dose regimen bled excessively. The thromboembolic rates were 42% in the patients receiving 10 mg, 9% in the patients receiving 15 mg, and 10% in the patients receiving 20 mg. Although the numbers are small, the reduced rates of thromboembolism compare favorably with those reported for low molecular weight heparins when used prophylactically. The results of these 2 studies support further evaluations of the use of hirudin and hirulog for the prevention of venous thrombosis in patients undergoing major orthopedic surgery.

B. TREATMENT OF PATIENTS WITH VENOUS THROMBOSIS

Two small published trials of direct thrombin inhibitors, one with hirulog and one with hirudin, for the treatment of patients with venous thrombosis have been reported.[14,15] The purpose of the first study was to determine whether a single injection of hirulog, which prolongs the aPTT twofold, produces a sustained inhibition of the increased activation of coagulation present in patients with calf DVT at the time of diagnosis. Ten patients with venographically-demonstrated calf vein thrombosis received a single injection of hirulog, either 1.0 mg/kg subcutaneously or 0.6 mg/kg as a 15 minute intravenous infusion. Both hirulog regimens produced a more than twofold prolongation of the aPTT. Prothrombin fragment (F1+2) levels, used as an index of thrombin generation, were measured before as well as 6 and 24 hours post-hirulog administration. Patients were followed with non-invasive tests to detect thrombus extension into the proximal veins.

There was a significant reduction in the levels of endogenous F1+2 with both regimens, 6 hours after hirulog (Table 3). The F1+2 levels at 24 hours were significantly higher than the 6-hour post-hirulog results. One patient developed thrombus extension into the popliteal vein and was treated with conventional anticoagulants. Therefore, the regimens of hirulog used in this study produced incomplete and temporary suppression of F1+2. Complete and permanent inhibition of thrombin generation by hirulog in patients with calf vein thrombosis may require multiple subcutaneous injections and/or prolonged intravenous infusion. Complete inhibition of F1+2 elevation may not be achieved if prothrombinase in the thrombus, rather than new prothrombinase, accounts for most of the thrombin generation.

The second study was an open pilot design, which evaluated the efficacy of intravenous recombinant hirudin in 10 patients with proximal venous thrombosis.[15] Hirudin was given as an intravenous bolus of 0.07 mg/kg, followed by an infusion of 0.05 mg/kg/hour for 5 days. Then, low molecular weight heparin and acenocoumarol were administered, the latter for 3 months. None of the patients died or suffered thromboembolic recurrence or bleeding during the trial. Serial lung scanning and venography demonstrated that there was no deterioration of the patients during the study. The aPTT ratio ranged between 1.2 and 2.8. Although the number is small, these results suggest that further evaluation of hirudin for the treatment of patients with venous thrombosis is warranted.

C. TREATMENT OF PATIENTS WITH UNSTABLE ANGINA

Thrombus formation caused by rupture of an atherosclerotic plaque is important in the pathophysiology of unstable angina.[16] Heparin is efficacious in reducing the rate of symptom progression in patients with unstable angina, presumably due to its antithrombotic effects.[17] Two studies, one with hirulog and one with hirudin, have evaluated direct thrombin inhibitors in patients with unstable angina.[18,19] In the first study, a two-part dose-ranging study of patients with unstable angina was performed. In the first part of the study, 15 patients received an intravenous infusion of hirulog 0.02, 0.05, 0.1, 0.25, and 0.5 mg/kg/hour, each dose given over 15 minutes. There was significant reduction in fibrinopeptide A (FPA) as compared to baseline, seen during infusion of 0.25 mg/kg/hour. Therefore, this dose was

Table 3
A Phase 2 Study of Hirulog for the Treatment of Patients with Calf Deep Vein Thrombosis

F1+2 Data In Patients Treated With Hirulog 1.0 mg/kg Subcutaneously

	F1+2 Levels (nmol/L)		
Pt #	Pre	6 hrs Post	24 hrs Post
1	2.4	1.5	2.1
2	1.9	1.2	1.2
3	2.0	1.5	1.3
4	2.0	1.4	1.8
5	2.7	1.8	2.2

(mean 2.20 ± 0.34; 1.48 ± 0.22; 1.72 ± 0.45 ± SD)

F1+2 Data In Patients Treated With Hirulog 0.6 mg/kg Intravenously

	F1+2 Levels (nmol/L)		
Pt #	Pre	6 hrs Post	24 hrs Post
1	1.4	0.9	1.4
2	2.2	1.8	3.7
3	1.8	1.7	N/A
4	1.7	1.7	2.2
5	1.7	1.4	1.6

(mean 1.76 ± 0.29; 1.50 ± 0.37; 2.23 ± 1.04 ± SD)

N/A, not available.

used as the starting dose for the second part of the study. The dose escalations in the second part of the study were made when 2 treatment failures occurred with the intention of achieving a 95% success rate. Five patients received 0.25 mg/kg/hour and 14 received 0.5 mg/kg/hour before the 2 failures occurred. Failure was observed in only 1 of 21 patients who received 1.0 mg/kg/hour (success rate of 95%). In the highest dose regimen, the mean aPTT was 98 seconds. FPA levels decreased with all treatment regimens, but this effect was most consistent with the highest treatment regimen. No deaths, myocardial infarctions, or bleeding complications occurred.

In the second study[19], patients with ischemic pain at rest, an abnormal electrocardiogram, and a baseline angiogram indicating

≥60% stenosis of a culprit coronary artery or saphenous vein graft with visual appearance of thrombus, were enrolled. The patients were randomized to one of two treatment regimens of heparin (given in a dose to prolong the aPTT to 65-90 seconds or to 90-110 seconds) or one of four doses of hirudin (0.05, 0.10, 0.20, or 0.30 mg/kg/hour infusion preceded by a bolus of 0.15 mg/kg, 0.3 mg/kg, 0.6 mg/kg, or 0.6 mg/kg, respectively), in a dose-escalating protocol. Three patients received a 0.9 mg/kg bolus of hirudin followed by an infusion of 0.3 mg/kg/hour, but this treatment regimen was discontinued because of significant bleeding. After 72 to 120 hours of the study drug, a repeat coronary angiogram was obtained and the paired study underwent quantitative analysis. The primary end-point was change in the average cross-sectional area of the culprit lesion. Other efficacy end-points also involved changes in culprit lesion dimensions and TIMI flow grade. Overall, the 116 patients treated with hirudin tended to show more improvement than the 50 patients receiving heparin relative to the primary efficacy variable, the average cross-sectional area ($p = 0.08$), as well as minimal cross-sectional area ($p = 0.028$), minimal luminal diameter ($p = 0.029$), and percent diameter stenosis ($p = 0.07$). Major bleeding occurred in less than 5% of patients in all treatment arms, and was always secondary to a procedure. No spontaneous major bleeding occurred. There were no deaths during the study, and the rates of myocardial infarction and recurrent angina were not significantly different between the hirudin- and the heparin-treated patients.

These studies suggest that hirulog and hirudin are potentially useful in managing patients with unstable angina, and that further evaluations of these agents in large-scale clinical trials may be warranted.

D. PREVENTION OF REOCCLUSION OF THE CORONARY ARTERIES AFTER ANGIOPLASTY OR THROMBOLYTIC THERAPY

Heparin has been used for several years for the prevention of reocclusion of coronary arteries after angioplasty or thrombolytic therapy. In spite of the use of heparin, there are still clinically significant rates of abrupt closure after coronary angioplasty and reocclusion of coronary arteries after the use of thrombolytic therapy in patients with acute myocardial infarction.[4,5] There have been 3 published studies of direct thrombin inhibitors given for the prevention of reocclusion of the coronary arteries.[20-22] The first was a multicenter dose escalation study in which 291 patients undergoing elective coronary angioplasty (and pretreated with 325 mg aspirin daily) were enrolled in sequential groups to receive intravenously administered hirulog as follows: group 1, a 0.15 mg/kg bolus followed by an infusion of 0.6 mg/kg/hour (54 patients); group 2, a 0.25 mg/kg bolus followed by an infusion of 1.0 mg/kg/hour (53 patients); group 3, a 0.35 mg/kg bolus followed by an infusion of 1.4 mg/kg/hour (44 patients); group 4, bolus 0.45 mg/kg followed by an infusion of 1.8 mg/kg/hour (74 patients); group 5, bolus 0.55 mg/kg followed by an infusion of 2.2 mg/kg/hour (54 patients). The hirulog infusion was maintained for 4 hours and the primary end-point was abrupt vessel closure within 24 hours of the initiation of the procedure. Abrupt vessel closure occurred in 18 patients (6.2%). By intention to treat analysis, the abrupt closure event rate for groups 1-3 was 11.3% compared with 3.9% for groups 4 and 5 ($p = 0.052$). There were no significant bleeding complications except in one patient in group 1 who required a 2-unit transfusion. A dose-response curve of aPTTs was seen and group 5 showed a fivefold prolongation in the aPTT ratio. This study demonstrates that hirulog may be safe and potentially efficacious in preventing abrupt vessel closure after coronary angioplasty (groups 4 and 5).

Two other studies (published as abstracts) have used direct thrombin inhibitors to prevent reocclusion following thrombolytic therapy in patients with acute myocardial infarction.[21,22] The first study, the TIMI 5 Trial, was a randomized, open-label dose-ranging trial of hirudin versus heparin given in conjunction with front-loaded tissue plasminogen activator and aspirin to 214 patients with acute myocardial infarction.[21] Patients received either heparin (in a dose adjusted to prolong the aPTT to 65-90 seconds) or hirudin (given as a bolus, followed by a constant infusion at 1 of 4 doses: 1) bolus of 0.15 mg/kg followed by an infusion of 0.05 mg/kg/hour; 2) bolus of 0.10 mg/kg followed by an infusion of 0.1 mg/kg/hour; 3) bolus of 0.3 mg/kg followed by an infusion of 0.1 mg/kg/hour; 4) bolus of 0.6 mg/kg followed by an infusion of 0.2 mg/kg/hour.

Patients underwent angiography at 90 minutes, and again at 18-36 hours if the culprit vessel was patent at 90 minutes. The late angiogram results showed that hirudin treatment in 105 patients significantly increased the rates of TIMI flow 2 or 3 (99% versus 93% in the heparin-treated groups) and significantly lowered the rates of reocclusion (1% versus 7% in the heparin-treated patients, $n = 60$). Spontaneous hemorrhage was observed in 3% of patients in both treatment arms.

In the second study, hirulog was compared to heparin as adjunctive therapy to streptokinase in 42 patients with acute myocardial infarction.[22] The patients received aspirin (325 mg) and streptokinase (1.5 million U) over 1 hour. Then, the patients were randomized to receive hirulog, 0.5 mg/kg/hour for 12 hours followed by 0.1 mg/kg/hour for 84 hours ($n = 28$); or heparin, 1,000 U/hour, which was adjusted to double the aPTT (n = 14). The primary end-point was TIMI grade 2 to 3 angiographic patency of the infarct-related artery. There was a significantly higher patency rate in the hirulog-treated patients (86%) than in the heparin-treated patients (43%). There was one systemic hemorrhage in the hirulog treatment group (4%) compared to three systemic hemorrhages in the heparin treatment group (21%).

E. SUMMARY OF STUDIES AND FUTURE PERSPECTIVES

These studies suggest that the direct thrombin inhibitors have considerable potential for use in the prevention and treatment of venous and arterial thrombosis. For each of the indications discussed above, hirudin and hirulog appear potentially safe, and efficacious regimens for evaluation in Phase 3 studies have been described. Another potential advantage of these agents is the apparent lack of thrombocytopenia associated with their use, presumably due to a lack of immunologic cross-reactivity with heparin. Consequently, it is possible that these direct thrombin inhibitors will be useful in patients with heparin-induced thrombocytopenia. These studies also provide direct evidence that thrombin has a pivotal role in the pathogenesis of arterial and venous thrombosis because the direct thrombin inhibitors only inactivate thrombin.

Three important issues remain outstanding. First, definitive proof of the efficacy and safety of these agents must be obtained from larger randomized and blinded clinical trials. Second, it is unclear whether other direct anti-thrombins (which are currently being developed) will be superior clinically to the currently available agents. Third, the potential improvement in efficacy and safety associated with the use of these agents must be sufficiently significant to justify the inevitable increased expense as compared to the efficacy and safety versus cost of currently available agents.

REFERENCES

1. **Hirsh, J.** Oral anticoagulant drugs. *N Engl J Med*, 324, 1865, 1991.
2. **Hirsh, J.** Heparin. *N Engl J Med*, 324, 1565, 1991.
3. **Hirsh, J., Levine, M.** Prevention of venous thrombosis in patients undergoing major orthopaedic surgical procedures. *Br J Clin Pract*, 65, 2, 1989.
4. **Collen, D., Lijnen, H.R.** Basic and clinical aspects of fibrinolysis and thrombolysis. *Blood*, 78, 3114, 1991.
5. **Lincoff, A.M., Popma, J.J., Ellis, S.G., Hacker, J.A., Topol, E.J.** Abrupt vessel closure complicating coronary angioplasty: Clinical,

angiographic and therapeutic profile. *J Am Coll Cardiol*, 19, 926, 1992.

6. **Weitz, J.I., Hudoba, M., Massel, D., Maraganore, J., Hirsh, J.** Clot-bound thrombin is protected from inhibition by heparin-antithrombin III but is susceptible to inactivation by antithrombin III-independent inhibitors. *J Clin Invest*, 86, 385, 1990.
7. **Hogg, P.J., Jackson, C.M.** Fibrin monomer protects thrombin from inactivation by heparin-antithrombin III: Implications for heparin efficacy. *Proc Natl Acad Sci USA*, 86, 3619, 1989.
8. **Agnelli, G., Renga, C., Weitz, J.I., Nenci, G.G., Hirsh, H.** Sustained antithrombotic activity of hirudin after its plasma clearance: Comparison with heparin. *Blood*, 80, 960, 1992.
9. **Ofosu, F.A., Agnelli, G., Hirsh, J.** New thrombin inhibitors: Mode of action, experimental findings and clinical potential. In: *Rec Adv Haemat*. Hoffbrand, V. and Brenner, M.K. (eds), Churchill Livingstone, London, 1992, Vol 6, pp 45.
10. **Ofosu, F.A.** A personal communication, 1994.
11. **Ginsberg, J.S., Hirsh, J., Gent, M., MacKinnon, B., Turpie, A.G.G., Levine, M.N., Powers, P., Weitz, J.I., Findlen, K., Neemeh, J., Buller, H., Adelman, B., Maraganore, J., Fox., I.** A phase II study of hirulog in the prevention of venous thrombosis after major hip or knee surgery. *Circ*, 86, I-409, 1992.
12. **Green, D.** Prevention of thromboembolism after spinal cord injury. *Semin Thromb Hemost*, 17, 347, 1991.
13. **Eriksson, B.I., Kalebo, P., Lindbratt, S., Ekman, S., Close, P.** Is direct thrombin inhibition with hirudin a safe prophylaxis of thromboembolic complications after hip replacement?, *Circ*, 86, 1634, 1992.
14. **Ginsberg, J.S., Nurmohamed, M.T., Gent, M., MacKinnon, B., Stevens, P., Weitz, J., Maraganore, J., Hirsh, J.** Effects on thrombin generation of single injections of hirulog in patients with calf vein thrombosis, Unpublished data.
15. **Parent, F., Bridey, F., Dreyfus, M., Musset, D., Grimon, G., Duroux, P., Meyer, D., Simonneau, G.** Treatment of severe venous thrombo-embolism with intravenous hirudin (HBW 023): An open pilot study. *Thromb Haemost*, 70, 386, 1993.
16. **Davies, M.J., Thomas, A.C.** Plaque fissuring the cause of acute myocardial infarction, sudden ischemic death, and crescendo angina. *Br Heart J*, 53, 363, 1981.
17. **Theroux, P., Ouimet, H., McCans, J., Latour, J-G., Joly, P., Levy, G., Pelletier, E., Juneau, M., Stasiak, J., de Guise, P., Pelletier, G.B., Rinzler, D., Waters, D.D.** Aspirin, heparin, or both to treat acute unstable angina. *N Engl J Med*, 319, 1105, 1988.

18. **Lidon, R-M., Theroux, P., Juneau, M., Adelman, B., Maraganore, J.** Initial experience with a direct antithrombin, hirulog, in unstable angina. Anticoagulant, antithrombotic, and clinical effects. *Circ*, 88, 1495, 1993.
19. **Topol, E.J., Fuster, V., Harrington, R.A., Califf, R.M., Kleiman, N.S., Kereiakes, D.J., Cohen, M., Chapekis, A., Gold, H.K., Tannenbaum M.A., Rao, A.K., Debowey, D., Schwartz, D., Henis, M., Chesebro, J.** Recombinant hirudin for unstable angina pectoris. A multicenter, randomized angiographic trial, Unpublished data.
20. **Topol, E.J., Bonan, R., Jewitt, D., Sigwart, U., Kakkar, V.V., Rothman, M., de Bono, D., Ferguson, J., Willerson, J.T., Strony, J., Ganz, P., Cohen, M., Raymond, R., Fox, I., Maraganore, J., Adelman, B.** Use of a direct antithrombin, hirulog, in place of heparin during coronary angioplasty. *Circ*, 87, 1622, 1993.
21. **Cannon, C.P., McCabe, C.H., Henry, T.D., Rogers, W.J., Schweiger, M., Gibson, R.S., Anderson, J.L., Williams, D.O., Braunwald, E.** Hirudin reduces reocclusion compared to heparin following thrombolysis in acute myocardial infarction: Results of the TIMI 5 trial. *J Am Coll Cardiol*, 21, 136A, 1993.
22. **Lidon, R-A., Theroux, P., Bonan, R., Lesperance, J., Maragnore, J., Adelman, B., Waters, D.** Hirulog as adjunctive therapy to streptokinase in acute myocardial infarction. *J Am Coll Cardiol*, 21, 419A, 1993.
23. **Young, E., Prins, M., Levine, M.N., Hirsh, J.** Heparin binding to plasma proteins, an important mechanism for heparin resistance. *Thromb Haemost*, 67, 639, 1992.

Chapter 6

DEVELOPMENT AND RATIONALE FOR USE OF ANTI-THROMBINS IN ARTERIAL THROMBOSIS

Stephanie J. Brister, Frederick A. Ofosu and Michael R. Buchanan

I. INTRODUCTION

Fissuring or rupture of an atherosclerotic plaque in a coronary artery, with subsequent formation of a mural or occlusive thrombus, is fundamental to the development of acute ischemic symptoms.[1-3] Plaques which are prone to rupture are composed of a crescentic mass of lipids separated from the vessel lumen by a fibrous cap. They are relatively soft with an eccentric accumulation of cholesterol.[4] Shear rates, acute changes in coronary pressure or tone, and bending and twisting can all contribute to plaque rupture.[5] This deep vessel wall injury results in exposure of the circulating blood to collagen, lipids, and other elements of vessel wall to blood, thereby facilitating thrombin generation and thrombin deposition.[6] Platelet and fibrinogen deposition onto an injured vessel wall *in vivo* are thrombin dependent and occur within minutes of deep arterial injury, establishing the nidus of a forming thrombus.[7] Spontaneous lysis can occur, but alternatively any residual thrombus can persist. Acute coronary syndromes may result from the protrusion of a residual mural thrombus, which causes a decrease of luminal diameter and an increase in the shear stress on the vessel wall. In addition, the residual thrombus remains highly thrombogenic and can promote total vessel occlusion and result in clinical symptoms.[5]

Thrombin is generated via the intrinsic and extrinsic coagulation systems.[8,9] Platelets, white cells and smooth muscle cells provide binding sites for the assembly of the prothrombinase complex.[9] thrombinase is the prothrombin activation complex composed of Factors Xa and Va and calcium, and is assembled on phospholipids of cell surfaces such as activated platelets and smooth muscle cells.[9-11] Following deep arterial injury, tissue factor becomes available on the cell surface to interact with Factor VII to form VIIa, which then activates Factor X to initiate prothrombin formation. The rate of thrombin generation by prothrombinase is 278,000 times faster than the rate achieved by free Factor Xa. Thrombin has multiple actions which include conversion of fibrinogen to fibrin (an important constituent in venous thrombi), activation of Factor XIII to Factor XIIIa (which cross-links fibrin, thereby stabilizing the thrombus), activation

0-8493-7649-1/95/$0.00+$.50

of Factor V to Factor Va, and activation of platelets (see Chapter 1).[8] The last action of thrombin is probably pivotal in the pathogenesis of arterial thrombosis.[7]

II. THE PROTHROMBOTIC STATE

Increased levels of circulating thrombin are present in clinical situations and are thought to reflect increased risk for venous and arterial thrombosis. Ardissimo et al.[12] found that the 24-hour urinary excretion of Fibrinopeptide A (a measure of thrombin activity) was higher in patients with unstable angina and angiographically documented intracoronary thrombi than the urinary levels of Fibrinopeptide A in patients with unstable angina but without documented thrombi. Gulba et al.[13] treated 55 patients with urokinase-preactivated prokinase or tissue plasminogen activator for acute myocardial infarction. The patients underwent coronary angiography at 90 minutes and 24-36 hours after commencing the thrombolytic therapy. Plasma fibrinopeptide A, D-dimer and thrombin-antithrombin III (TAT) complex levels which were measured varied according to the response to treatment. For example, the TAT levels decreased in those patients with persistent patency, and increased in those patients with unsuccessful thrombolysis or early reocclusion. Fondevilla et al.[14] demonstrated that TAT and the prothrombin fragment F1+2 (F1+2) levels measured during angiography and percutaneous transluminal angioplasty (PTCA) were elevated during and after the procedure. Moreover, Gill et al.[15] demonstrated that TAT and F1+2 levels increased even further in patients undergoing PTCA when the post-PTCA heparin infusion was stopped. These studies suggest that these cardiac patients are at risk of further thrombotic events. Brister et al.[16] and Boisclair et al.[17] reported that thrombin generation increases significantly during the course of cardiac surgery despite administration of high doses of heparin. Thus, data from a variety of clinical settings suggest that an amplified systemic response of thrombin generation can persist following the initial generation of thrombin in response to vessel wall injury or exposure to a foreign surface. This additional thrombin generation may enhance the risk of thrombotic events in these patients. The observations that thrombin generation increases following cessation of heparin therapy after PTCA and cardiac surgery, also suggest that the initiating stimuli for thrombin generation remain active and require further antithrombotic treatment to minimize the risk for post-procedural thrombotic events.

The therapeutic approaches which have been used in the treatment of arterial thrombosis include anticoagulants, anti-fibrinolytics, anti-platelet agents and anti-thrombins. In this chapter we will focus on the anti-thrombins.

III. REGULATION OF THE PROTHROMBOTIC STATE

A. HEPARIN

Heparin, a naturally occurring glycosaminoglycan, catalyzes the inhibition of thrombin and other coagulant enzymes by antithrombin III (ATIII). It is currently the most commonly used antithrombotic drug. Telford and Wilson[18] published the first randomized study demonstrating a benefit of heparin in patients with unstable angina who had suffered a non Q-wave myocardial infarction. Theroux et al.[19] also demonstrated that the incidence of myocardial infarction or death decreased from 11.9% in placebo-control patients to 0.8% in heparin-treated patients. In contrast, Wallentin et al.[20] found no significant decrease in myocardial infarction with heparin. The latter study however, included a low risk population. In addition, no other anti-platelet or anti-thrombin drug was given to the heparin-treated patients after 5 days, the time when heparin was discontinued. Consequently, there may have been a rebound thrombotic effect which contributed to an increase in the event rate in that patient group. A rebound effect has been described in similar clinical situations by other investigators.[14,15] In Italy, 58 hospitalized patients with recurrent ischemia in the previous 24 hours were first randomized into stage 1 of a 2-stage trial. In stage 1, the patients were administered either 1) a heparin infusion [to prolong the activated partial thromboplastin time (aPTT) 1.5 to 2 times the control] or 2) a heparin bolus (6,000 U IV q.6.h.), or 3) aspirin (325 mg daily). The end-points measured were the presence of transient ST-segment depression during a 72-hour Holter monitoring period and the presence of angina during the following 4 days. The intravenous infusion of heparin was the only treatment which decreased significantly the incidence of recurrent ischemia.[21] However, even in the studies which show benefit with heparin, a significant proportion of the patients continued to have unstable angina or proceeded to infarction despite the heparin therapy. Consequently heparin may not be the most efficacious anti-thrombin in this setting.

Heparin has both anti-Factor Xa and anti-thrombin catalytic activities. Buchanan et al.[22] have clearly demonstrated that inhibition of venous thrombus formation is achieved more readily with agents that catalyze thrombin inhibition than with agents which enhance Factor Xa inhibition. Heras et al.[23] demonstrated that despite the greater anti-Factor Xa to anti-thrombin ratios of low molecular weight heparin fractions, these agents do not significantly reduce platelet or fibrinogen deposition in experimental arterial thrombosis. Thus, accelerated thrombin inhibition provides a more reliable antithrombotic effect than accelerated Factor Xa inhibition. These data also suggest that heparin is not the ideal anti-thrombin in arterial thrombosis. Hogg and Jackson[24] demonstrated that the ability of heparin to catalyze thrombin inhibition by ATIII becomes impaired when the thrombin is bound to fibrin *in vitro*. Similar results were found when thrombin was bound to extracellular vascular components *in vitro*[6], to freshly formed thrombi *in vivo*[25] or in deep arterial injury in a pig model.[7] In summary, thrombin bound to fibrin is resistant to inhibition by heparin/ATIII. It appears that heparin must bind not only to ATIII at a high affinity site, but also to thrombin at an anionic exosite (see Chapter 2). The thrombin exosite to which heparin binds may overlap the site to which thrombin binds fibrin.

When used clinically, heparin is thought to catalyze effectively the inhibition of circulating thrombin. It has become increasingly apparent that the surface- or clot-bound thrombin (which is resistant to inhibition by heparin/ATIII) remains active and stimulates the generation of further thrombin. The situation is clearly illustrated in the setting of cardiopulmonary bypass surgery. High doses of heparin (300 units/kg) are required to prevent thrombus formation in the circuit, but these doses do not prevent the generation of high concentrations of thrombin during the procedure[16,17]; the heparin only appears to control the clinical sequelae of it. Thrombin bound to the surface of the extracorporeal circuit may be precipitating the ongoing generation of the thrombin and creating a prothrombotic environment.[16,17,26] In acute coronary syndromes or following PTCA, the thrombin on the injured vessel surface is likely to remain active and to contribute to the thrombotic events which occur following cessation of heparin.

B. HIRUDIN AND PPACK

Recognition of these phenomena has led to the development of other anti-thrombins which inactivate thrombin directly or catalyze the inhibition of thrombin by heparin cofactor II (HCII). Hirudin, a direct thrombin inhibitor, binds to thrombin (Ki $\leq 10^{-15}$ M) to displace thrombin from its binding site on platelets and possibly from binding sites on other tissue.[27-29] Weitz et al.[30,31] have demonstrated that the synthetic thrombin inhibitor D-phenylalany-L-propyl-L-arginyl chloromethyl ketone (PPACK) and hirudin inhibit both fluid-phase and clot-bound thrombin equally.

In the TIMI 5 Trial, hirudin was compared to heparin in an open label, dose-ranging trial in 214 patients with recent myocardial infarction.[32] Both drugs were administered in conjunction with tissue plasminogen activator and aspirin. Patients received either heparin (the dose was adjusted to maintain a prolonged aPTT of 65-90 seconds) or 1 of 4 doses of hirudin given as a bolus, followed by an infusion. Angiography was performed at 90 minutes and again 18-36 hours later if the culprit vessel was patent at 90 minutes. Hirudin treatment significantly increased the rates of TIMI flow 2 or 3 (99% in hirudin patients versus 93% in heparin patients) and lowered the rates of reocclusion from 7% in the heparin-treated patients to 1% in the hirudin-treated patients. The incidence of spontaneous hemorrhage was 3% in both drugs. The TIMI 6 Trial was a randomized, open label, pilot study to evaluate the safety of hirudin versus heparin when administered in conjunction with streptokinase and aspirin in 193 patients with acute myocardial infarction. Patients received either a 5-day course of heparin (n = 71, 5000 U bolus, followed by a constant infusion to achieve an aPTT of 65-90 seconds, or a constant infusion of 1 of 3 doses of hirudin (n = 55, 0.15 mg/kg bolus + 0.05 mg/kg/hr infusion; n = 31, 0.3 bolus + 0.1 mg/kg/hr infusion; or n = 36, 0.6 bolus + 0.2 mg/kg/hr infusion). There were non-significant trends towards a lower incidence of death and cardiac events in the patients treated with the two higher doses of hirudin, as compared to the incidence of death and cardiac events in the patients treated with heparin. The incidence of major hemorrhage was equivalent (5-6%) in the heparin treated patients and the hirudin-treated patients at any dose.[33] In the ongoing TIMI 9 Trial, a double blind trial of hirudin versus heparin may help us to conclude whether hirudin is more effective than heparin in this clinical situation.

Chesebro et al.[34] compared the effectiveness of recombinant hirudin (in a dose-escalating protocol) to heparin at 2 doses (targeted to prolong the aPTT to 65-90 seconds or 90-110 seconds) in patients with unstable angina. Angiography was performed at the outset of the study and 78-108 hours later. Primary end-points were changes in culprit lesion dimensions and TIMI flow grade. The change in cross-sectional area for heparin (0.08 mm^2) was less than the change seen with hirudin (0.31 mm^2), but this difference was not significant ($p = 0.08$). The incidence of myocardial infarction however, was lower in the hirudin-treated patients (2.6%) as compared to the heparin-treated patients (8%).

Hirulog, [D-Phe-Pro-Arg-Pro-$(Gly)_4$-Asn-Gly-Asp-Phe-Glu-Glu-Ile-Pro-Glu-Glu-Tyr-Leu] is a bifunctional anti-thrombin, combining the catalytic site binding ligand, D-Phe-Pro-Arg, with the hirudin tail, which has high affinity for a fibrinogen binding exosite of thrombin.[36] The fourth residue, Pro, was added to minimize cleavage of the inhibitor at the third residue. *In vitro* hirulog inhibits clot-bound thrombin more effectively than heparin.[36] Hirulog has also been administered clinically. In one study, 55 patients with unstable angina were entered in an acute dose-escalating study (Phase 1). Then, the sustained anticoagulant and antithrombotic effects of the drug were assessed during a 72-hour infusion (Phase 2).[37] Successful control of symptoms occurred in all but one patient who received a dose of hirulog 1 mg/kg/hr. The Fibrinopeptide A levels decreased with all hirulog doses but more consistently with a dose of greater than 1 mg/kg/hr. The success rate in preventing recurrent chest pain was 87.5%, and no deaths or myocardial infarctions occurred. In addition, there was no significant bleeding during the treatment period.

Topol et al.[38] reported on the use of hirulog in 291 patients undergoing elective PTCA. This study was also an open label dose-finding study in which patients were administered 1 of 5 doses of hirulog, given as a bolus, followed by an infusion during PTCA instead of the conventional heparin dose. In addition, all patients were pre-treated with 325 mg of aspirin given orally. The acute closure rate in patients receiving hirulog (bolus 0.35 mg/kg; infusion 1.8 mg/kg/hr) was 11.3%. Only one patient required a blood transfusion, but it should be noted that the hemoglobin levels fell ≥2 g/dl in 18-37% of the patients in all hirulog-treated groups.

These studies demonstrate that direct thrombin inhibitors may be useful alternatives to heparin in various clinical settings of arterial thrombosis. For example, Fibrinopeptide A levels decrease in at least one clinical situation, namely, in unstable angina.[36] Elevated Fibrinopeptide A levels are associated with high levels of thrombin generation.[12] Theoretically, therefore, since the direct thrombin inhibitors readily inactivate both clot-bound and free thrombin, they should be able to prevent further thrombin-dependent thrombin production. However, to date, the appropriate therapeutic doses of these agents to achieve such an effect have not been determined. Moreover, the aPTT is prolonged when hirudin and hirulog are given in doses shown to have some clinical effect. Thus, it still is not clear whether patients treated with these direct thrombin inhibitors are at the same risk of bleeding as when treated with heparin. Certainly, the current clinical studies suggest that the incidence of hemorrhagic complications is comparable to heparin. This risk may increase even further if the dose of these agents has to be increased to achieve a therapeutic benefit rather than a prophylactic benefit, similar to heparin therapy.

C. HCII-DEPENDENT THROMBIN INHIBITORS

Heparin cofactor II (HCII) is a second endogenous inhibitor of thrombin.[39] Dermatan sulfate is a naturally occurring glycosaminoglycan found in the blood vessel wall[40] which catalyzes thrombin inhibition by HCII. Dermatan sulfate also catalyzes the inhibition of fibrin-bound thrombin as effectively as it catalyzes the inhibition of free thrombin (see Chapter 4).[41,42] In addition, dermatan sulfate appears to induce less bleeding in experimental animals than heparin, in marked contrast to the direct thrombin inhibitors.[43] Ryan et al. and others[44,45] have demonstrated that dermatan sulfate can be used effectively as an anticoagulant in patients undergoing hemodialysis. Others have reported that dermatan sulfate also prevents DVT in patients undergoing elective orthopedic surgery.[46-48] To date, however, dermatan sulfate has not been evaluated clinically in arterial thrombosis, but there is considerable data in animal studies which suggest that it could be an effective therapeutic agent. Van Ryn-McKenna et al.[49] demonstrated that a constant infusion of dermatan sulfate prevented fibrin accretion onto the surface of a thrombus more effectively than a constant infusion of heparin in a rabbit model of thrombosis. Additionally, they reported that dermatan sulfate facilitates tPA-induced thrombolysis more effectively than heparin.[50] In fact, when rabbits were administered heparin with tPA, thrombolysis was impaired as compared to the thrombolysis achieved with tPA alone. In contrast, when dermatan sulfate was administered with tPA, thrombolysis increased. Brister et al.[26] recently reported that the enhanced prothrombin turnover (a measure of thrombin generation and activity) seen during cardiopulmonary bypass in pigs is also blocked when dermatan sulfate is used as the anticoagulant instead of heparin. These investigators and others previously demonstrated that thrombin is generated during cardiopulmonary bypass in humans undergoing elective cardiac surgery despite the patients receiving high dose heparin.[16,17] In addition Buchanan et al.[51] have reported that dermatan sulfate when given acutely inhibits chronic vessel wall hyperplasia whereas heparin does not, using a rabbit model of arterial vessel wall hyperplasia. This latter study re-emphasizes the need to inhibit surface-bound thrombin at the time of injury or clot formation to prevent effectively both the immediate sequelae of thrombotic events and the long-term chronic sequelae of vessel wall hyperplasia.[51]

IV. CONCLUSION

Thrombin bound to an injured vessel wall or to a thrombus within the vessel wall lumen plays an integral role in the initiation and propagation of arterial thrombosis. This recognition has led to the utilization of anti-thrombins as a therapeutic approach to prevent or treat this process. While heparin and direct thrombin inhibitors have been shown to have some clinical benefits, bleeding-related side-effects occur with a small but consistent frequency. The direct anti-thrombins appear to inhibit surface-bound thrombin more effectively than heparin. The clinical effect of HCII-dependent agents should at least equal that of the direct thrombin inhibitors. Animal data suggest bleeding side-effects should be less. Their actual role in clinical therapeutics, however, remains to be defined although preliminary studies suggest they have a place in antithrombotic therapy.

REFERENCES

1. **Davies, M.J., Thomas, A.C.** Plaque fissuring cause of acute myocardial infarction, sudden ischemic death and crescendo angina. *Br Heart J* 53, 363, 1985.
2. **Falk, E.** Plaque rupture with severe pre-existing stenosis precipitating çoronary thrombosis: Characteristics of coronary atherosclerotic plaques underlying fatal occlusive thrombi. *Br Heart J* 50, 127, 1983.
3. **Fuster, V., Stern, B., Ambrose, J.A., Badimon, L., Badimon, J.J., Chesebro, J.** Atherosclerotic plaque rupture and thrombosis: Evolving concepts. *Circ* (Suppl II) II-47, 1982.
4. **Richardson, P.D., Davies, J.M., Born, C.V.R.** Influence of plaque configuration and stress distribution in fissuring of coronary atherosclerotic plaques. *Lancet* 2, 941, 1989.
5. **Fuster, V., Stern, B., Ambrose, J.A., Badimon, L., Badimon, J.J., Chesebro, J.** Insights into the pathogenesis of acute ischemic syndromes. *Circ* 77, 1213, 1988.
6. **Bar-Shavit, R., Elder, D., Vlodavsky, I.** Binding of thrombin to subendothelial extracellular matrix. *J Clin Invest* 84, 1096, 1989.
7. **Heras, M., Chesebro, J.H., Webster, M.W.I., Mruk, J.S., Grill, D.E., Penny, W.J., Bowie, E.J.W., Badimen, L., Mayda Fester, V.** Hirudin, heparin and placebo during deep arterial injury in the pig. The in vivo role of thrombin in platelet-mediated thrombosis. *Circ* 82, 1476, 1990.
8. **Shuman, M.A.** Thrombin-cellular interaction. *Ann NY Acad Sci* 485, 228, 1986.
9. **Mann, K.G., Nesheim, M.E., Church, W.R., Haley, P., Kirshnaswamy, S.** Surface-dependent reactions of the vitamin-K dependent enzyme complexes. *Blood* 76, 1, 1990.
10. **Mann, K.G., Nesheim, M.E., Hibbard, L.S.** The role of factor V in the assembly of the prothrombinase complex. *Ann NY Acad Sci* 370, 378, 1981.
11. **Nesheim, M., Tracy, R.P., Mann, K.G.** "Clot speed" a mathematical simulation of the functional properties of prothrombinase. *J Biol Chem* 259, 1447, 1984.

12. **Ardissimo, P., Gamba, M.G., Merlini, P.A., Rolla, A., Barbiera, P., Demicheli, G., Testa, S., Bruno, N., Specchia, G.** Fibrinopeptide A excretion in urine: A marker of the cumulative thrombin activity in stable versus unstable angina patients. *Am J Cardiol* 86, 58B, 1991.
13. **Gulba, D.C., Barthels, M., Westhoff-Black, M., Jost, S., Rafflenbend, W., Daniel, W.G., Hecker, H., Lichtlen, P.R.** Increased thrombin levels during thrombolytic therapy in acute myocardial infarction. *Circ* 83, 937, 1991.
14. **Fondevilla, C.G., Gill, J.B., Brister, S.J., Holder, D.A., Ofosu, F.A., Buchanan, M.R.** Contrast media induces thrombin generation during PTCA. *Thromb Haemost* 69, 1014, 1993.
15. **Gill, J.B., Holder, D.A., Brister, S.J., Ofosu, F.A., Buchanan, M.R.** Thrombin generation post PTCA following the cessation of heparin infusion. *Can J Cardiol* 9(E), 84, 1993.
16. **Brister, S.J., Ofosu, F.A., Buchanan, M.R.** Thrombin generation during cardiac surgery: Is heparin the ideal anticoagulant? *Thromb Haemost* 70, 259, 1993.
17. **Boisclair, M.D., Lane, D.A., Philippou, H., Esnouf, P., Sheikh, S., Hunt, B., Smith. K.J.** Mechanisms of thrombin generation during surgery and cardiopulmonary bypass. *Thromb Haemost* 69, 1307, 1993.
18. **Telford, A.M., Wilson, C.** Trial of heparin versus atenolol in prevention of myocardial infarction in intermediate coronary syndrome. *Lancet* 1, 1225, 1981.
19. **Theroux, P., Ourmet, H., McCans, J., Latoin, J.G., Joly, P., Levy, G., Pelletier, E., Juneau, M., Staslak, J., de Guise, P., Pelletier, G.B., Ringler, D., Waters, P.D.** Aspirin, heparin or both to treat acute unstable angina. *N Engl J Med* 319, 1105, 1988.
20. **Wallentin, L.**, For the RISC study group of unstable coronary artery disease. Risk for myocardial infarction and death in a randomized placebo-controlled study. *Circ* 80 (Suppl II) II-419, 1989.
21. **Serneri, N., Gensini, G.F., Poggesi, L., Trotta, F., Moesti, P.A., Boddi, M., Leri, M., Margheri, M., Casolo, G.G., Bini, M., Rostagno, L., Carnovali, M., Abbate, R.** Effect of heparin, aspirin or alteplase in reduction of myocardial ischemia in refractory unstable angina. *Lancet* 335, 615, 1990.
22. **Buchanan, M.R., Boneu, B., Ofosu, F., Hirsh, J.** The relevant importance of the antithrombotic effects of heparin. *Blood* 65, 198, 1985.
23. **Heras, M., Chesebro, J.H., Webster, M.W.I., Mruk, J.S., Grill, D.E., Badimon, L., Fuster, V.** Antithrombotic efficacy of low

molecular weight heparin in deep arterial injury. *Arterioscler Thromb* 12, 250, 1992.
24. **Hogg, P.J., Jackson, C.M.** Fibrin monomer protects thrombin from inactivation by heparin-antithrombin III. Implications for heparin efficacy. *Proc Natl Acad Sci* 86, 619, 1989.
25. **Okwusidi, J.I., Falcone, M., Van-Ryn-McKenna, J., Hirsh, J., Ofosu, F.A., Buchanan, M.R.** In vivo catalysis of thrombin inhibition by antithrombin III or heparin co-factor II and antithrombotic effect. Differential effects of unfractionated heparin and dermatan sulfate. *Thromb Haemost Dis* 1, 77, 1990.
26. **Brister, S.J., Ofosu, F.A., Gianese, F., Heigenhauser, G.F., Buchanan, M.R.** Dermatan sulfate prevents prothrombin consumption during cardiopulmonary bypass more effectively than heparin. *Thromb Haemost* 69, 1256, 1993.
27. **Mao, S.J.T., Yates, M.T., Owen, T.J., Krstenansky, J.L.** Interaction of hirudin with thrombin: identification of a minimal binding domain of hirudin that inhibits clotting activity. *Biochem* 27, 8170, 1988.
28. **Tam, W.S., Fenton, J.W., Detwiler, T.C.** Dissociation of thrombin from platelets by hirudin. *J Biol Chem* 254, 8723, 1979.
29. **Stone, S.R., Hofsteenge, J.** Kinetics of the inhibition of thrombin by hirudin. *Biochem* 25, 4622, 1986.
30. **Weitz, J.I., Hudoba, M., Massel, D., Maraganore, J., Hirsh, J.** Clot-bound thrombin is protected from inhibition by heparin-antithrombin III but is susceptible to inactivation by antithrombin III-dependent inhibitors. *J Clin Invest* 86, 385, 1990.
31. **Massel, D.R., Hudoba, M., Weitz, J.I.** Clot-bound thrombin is protected from heparin inhibition: a potential mechanism for rethrombosis after lytic therapy. *Circ* 80 (Suppl II), II-420, 1989.
32. **Cannon, C.P., McCabe, C.H., Henry, T.D., Rogers, W.J., Schweizer, M., Gibson, R.S., Anderson, J.L., Williams, P.O., Braunwald, E.** Hirudin reduces reocclusion compared to heparin following thrombolysis in acute myocardial infarction: Results of the TIMI 5 Trial. *J Am Coll Cardiol* 21, 136A, 1993.
33. **Lee, V.L., MCCabe, C.H., Antman, E.M., Koch, M., Wilensky, R., Stringer, K., Hochman, J., Mueller, H.S., Henry, T.D., Kleiman, N., Steingart, R.M., Wasserman, H., Losordo, D., Ludbrook, P., Doorey, A., Rodriguez, S., Kennedy, P., Rogers, W.J., Williams, M.L., Smitherman, T.C., Gibson, R.S., Williams, J.T., Edwards, S., Henis, M., Braunwald, E.** For the TIMI 6 Investigators, *J Am Coll Cardiol* 788, 1994.
34. **Chesebro, J.H., Fuster, V., Califf, R.M., Harrington, R.A., Kleiman, N.S., Kereikes, D.J., Cohen, M., Chapekis, A., Gold, H.K., Bear, P., Rao, A.K., Debovey, D., Schwartz, D.,**

Heras, M., Topol, E.J. Recombinant hirudin for unstable angina: A pilot multicentre, randomized angiographic trial. *J Am Coll Cardiol* 363A, 944, 1994.

35. **Maraganore, J.M., Borriden, P., Jablonski, J., Ramachandran, K.L., Fenton, J.W., II.** Design and characterization of hirulog: a novel class of bivalent peptide inhibitors of thrombin. *Biochem* 29, 7095, 1990.
36. **Maraganore, J.M., Chao, B.H., Weitz, J.I., Hirsh, J.** Comparison of antithrombin activities of heparin and hirulog-1: basis for improved antithrombotic properties of direct thrombin inhibitors. *Thromb Haemost* 65, 506, 1991.
37. **Lidon, R.M., Theroux, P., Juneau, M., Adelman, B., Maraganore, J.** Initial experience with a direct antithrombin, hirulog, in unstable angina, anticoagulant, antithrombotic and clinical effects. *Circ* 88, 1495, 1988.
38. **Topol, E.J., Bonan, R., Jewitt, D., Sigwart, V., Kakkar, V.V., Rothman, M., de Bono, D., Ferguson, J., Weillerson, J.T., Strong, J., Ganz, P., Cohen, M.D., Ramond, R., Fox, I., Maraganore, J., Adelman, M.** Use of a direct anti-thrombin hirulog in place of heparin during coronary angioplasty. *Circ* 87, 1622, 1993.
39. **Tollefsen, D.M., Blank, M.K.** Detection of a new heparin-dependent inhibitor of thrombin in human plasma. *J Clin Invest* 68, 689, 1981.
40. **Murata, K.** Distribution of acidic glycosaminoglycans; lipids and water in normal human cerebral arteries of various ages. *Stroke* 16, 685, 1985.
41. **Okwusidi, J.I., Anvari, N., Kulczycky, M., Blajchman, M.A., Buchanan, M.R., Ofosu, F.A.** Fibrin moderates the catalytic action of heparin but not that of dermatan sulfate on thrombin inhibition in human plasma. *J Lab Clin Med* 117, 359, 1991.
42. **Bendayan, P., Boneu, B., Boccalon, P.** Dermatan sulfate is a more potent inhibitor of clot-bound thrombin than unfractionated and low molecular weight heparins. *Thromb Haemost* 69, 656, 1993.
43. **Fernandez, F., Van Ryn, J., Ofosu, F.A., Hirsh, J., Buchanan, M.R.** The hemorrhagic and antithrombotic effects of dermatan sulfate. *Br J Haematol* 64, 309, 1986.
44. **Ryan, K.E., Lane, D.A., Flynn, A., Ireland, H., Boisclair, M., Sheppard, J., Curtis, J.R.** Antithrombotic properties of dermatan sulfate (MF701) in hemodialysis for chronic renal failure. *Thromb Haemost* 68, 563, 1992.
45. **Nuimohamed, M.T., Knipscheer, H.C., Stevens, P., Krediet, P.T., Roggekamp, MC., Berekmans, R.J.,**

Ten Cate, J.W. Clinical experience with a new anticoagulant (dermatan sulfate) in chronic hemodialysis patients. *Clin Nephrol* 39, 166, 1992.

46. **Agnelli, C., Cosini, B., De Fillippo, P., Ranucci, V., Veschi, F., Langetti, M., Renga, C., Baizi, F., Gianese, F., Lupattelli, L., Rinenapoli, E., Nenci, G.G.** A randomized double blind, placebo controlled trial of dermatan sulfate for prevention of deep vein thrombosis in hip fracture. *Thromb Haemost* 67, 203, 1992.
47. **Prandoni, P., Meduri, F., Cuppini, S., Toniato, A., Zangrandi, F., Polistena, P., Gianese, F., Maffei-Faccioli, A.** Dermatan sulfate: a safe approach to prevention of post operative deep vein thrombosis. *Br J Surg* 79, 505, 1992.
48. **Cohen, A.T., Phillips, M.J., Edmondson, R.A., Melissou, E., Vaidynathan, I., Kakkar, V.V.** Dermatan sulfate for prophylaxis of deep vein thrombosis (DVT) in elective hip surgery: a double-binding trial. *Thromb Haemost* 69, 621, 1993.
49. **Van Ryn-McKenna, J., Brill-Edwards, P., Ofosu, F.A., Buchanan, M.R.** Inhibition of thrombus growth is achieved more effectively by catalysing thrombin inhibition by dermatan sulfate/heparin cofactor II than by heparin/antithrombin III. *Thromb Haemost* 65, 1391, 1991.
50. **Van Ryn-McKenna, J., Ofosu, F.A., Buchanan, M.R.** Dermatan sulfate increases tPA induced thrombolysis without increasing bleeding in rabbits. *Thromb Haemost* 65, 396, 1991.
51. **Buchanan, M.R., Brister, S.J., Laio, P., Warnke, C., Ofosu, F.A.** Effects of heparin and dermatan sulfate on injured vessel wall hyperplasia and vessel wall occlusion. *Thromb Haemost* 69, 950, 1993.

Chapter 7

PEDIATRIC THROMBOEMBOLISM: EPIDEMIOLOGY, PREVENTION AND TREATMENT

Maureen Andrew and Michèle David

I. INTRODUCTION

Deep venous thrombosis (DVT) and pulmonary embolism (PE) are well-recognized causes of morbidity and mortality in adults, and for this reason have been studied extensively. Compared to adults, DVT and PE are relatively rare events in children, but when present also cause significant morbidity and on occasion mortality. Because of the relatively low incidence of DVT/PE in children, the diagnostic and therapeutic approaches have been directly extrapolated from guidelines for adults. In order for this approach to be valid, several criteria need to be met, including a similar hemostatic system, natural history, and response to anticoagulant and thrombolytic agents in children and adults.

Studies of the relationship between age and hemostasis have documented profound effects of age on plasma concentrations of coagulation proteins[1-4] with secondary effects on the regulation of thrombin and plasmin.[4-6] A review of the French and English literature (1975 to 1992) and Canadian Registries of pediatric DVT/PE suggest that there are important differences in the epidemiology of DVT/PE in children compared to adults.[7,8] Both the developmental features of hemostasis and differences in the epidemiology of DVT/PE influence the response of children to anticoagulant and thrombolytic agents. Together these studies strongly suggest that optimal management of children with thromboembolic complications will differ significantly from adults. The following chapter reviews the evidence supporting the view that pediatric thromboembolism differs significantly from the adult, and that programs devoted to developing this speciality at a basic and clinical level are required. Arterial thrombosis and venous thrombosis outside of the deep venous system of the upper and lower extremity are not discussed.

II. THE RELATIONSHIP BETWEEN AGE AND THE OCCURRENCE OF DVT/PE

There is clear evidence that age is an important variable influencing the risk for thromboembolic complications within the adult population. The increasing risk for DVT/PE with age is important enough to

0-8493-7649-1/95/$0.00+$.50

influence recommendations for prophylactic anticoagulant regimens in high risk situations.[9-11] Estimates of the incidence of DVT/PE in children, from retrospective studies in single institutions, support the generally accepted view that the frequency of DVT/PE in children is significantly less than for adults.[12,13] The first analyses of the Canadian Registry of DVT/PE in children (ages 1 month to 18 years) reports an incidence of 0.07/10,000 children in Canada and an incidence of 5.3/10,000 in hospitalized children.[14] Comparable incidences of DVT/PE in the adult population have been estimated at 2.5 to 5.0% of the adult population.[15-17] There are other comparisons that can be made between children and adults that illustrate the lower risk of DVT/PE during childhood. **First,** a comprehensive review of the French and English literature indicates that only 308 cases of DVT/PE have been reported in children since 1975 compared to many thousands of cases in adult patients.[7] **Second,** in the absence of prophylactic anticoagulant therapy, the incidence of thromboembolic complications in adult patients following hip or knee replacement ranges between 40 and 60%.[18-20] Prophylactic anticoagulant therapy is not used in children following lower limb or scoliosis surgery and the rate of clinically apparent DVT/PE in this population is less than 1%.[21] **Third,** patients with a prethrombotic state due to a congenital deficiency of the major inhibitor of coagulation, antithrombin III (ATIII), rarely present with their first thromboembolic complication until early adulthood. In summary, children are protected from thromboembolic complications relative to adults.

III. MECHANISMS PROTECTING CHILDREN FROM THROMBOEMBOLIC COMPLICATIONS

Potential mechanisms responsible for protecting children from thromboembolic complications can be considered as: 1) enhanced thrombin regulation, 2) enhanced fibrinolysis, and 3) differences in platelet/vessel wall function and interaction. The following briefly summarizes the available information for these three possibilities.

A. THROMBIN REGULATION AND THROMBIN GENERATION

A decreased capacity to generate thrombin and/or an enhanced capacity to inhibit thrombin could provide protection from thromboembolic events. The capacity of plasmas from newborns to generate thrombin is decreased to 50% of adult values (Fig. 1).[3,22-24] The degree of impairment is similar to plasmas from adults receiving therapeutic amounts of coumadin or heparin.[22] Throughout the first 10 years of life, the capacity of plasmas to generate thrombin remains reduced to 80% of adult values.[25] In the presence of therapeutic

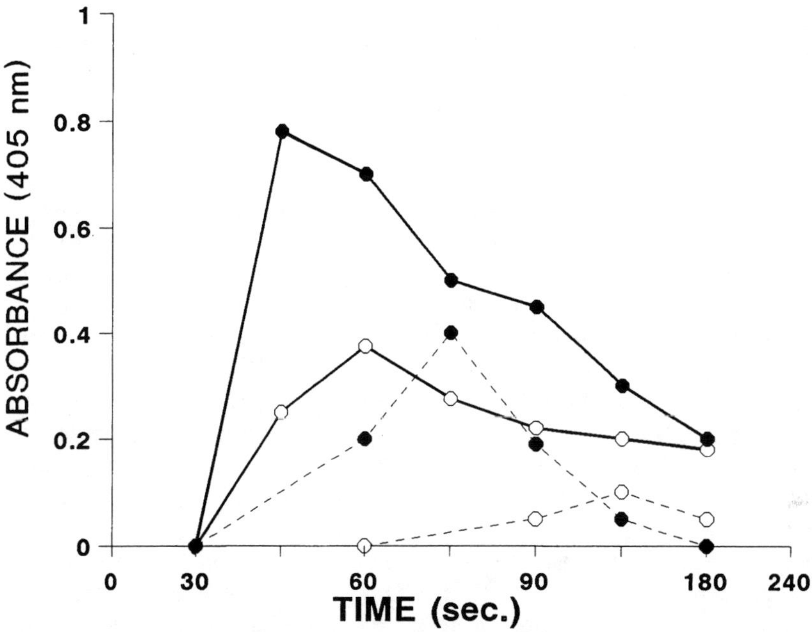

Figure 1. This figure shows that the thrombin-generating capacity of plasma from newborns, in the absence and presence of heparin, is significantly decreased compared to adult plasma. Adult ●—●; Adult:H ●---●; Newborn o—o; Newborn:H o---o.

concentrations of heparin, thrombin-generating capacity is abolished in newborn plasma and decreased to a greater extent in children's plasma compared to adult plasma.

At birth, plasma concentrations of the vitamin K dependant coagulant Factors II, VII, IX, and X; and the contact Factors XII, XI, prekallikrein (PK), and high molecular weight kininogen (HMWK) are approximately 50% of adult values.[1,2,26-29] Other coagulant proteins are present in concentrations similar to adults.[1,2,26-29] The levels of these proteins rapidly increase in the first weeks of life and are within the adult range of normal by 6 months.[1,2,29] However, average values of these coagulation proteins remain approximately 20% lower than adult values until the late teenage years.[4] When plasmas from infants and children were supplemented with purified coagulation proteins, the plasma concentration of prothrombin was the critically important determinant of the amount of thrombin generated.[3,25] These results are similar to those reported for plasmas from adults receiving warfarin therapy.[30] The decreased capacity to generate thrombin due to decreased levels of prothrombin, may provide one mechanism for protection from thromboembolic complications during childhood.

Thrombin converts fibrinogen to fibrin resulting in clot formation. At birth, fibrinogen is present in a "fetal" form, characterized by increased sialic acid content compared to adult fibrinogen.[31-33] The amino acid composition and the rate of release of fibrinopeptides A and B by thrombin are similar to adult fibrinogen.[31-33] These data do not support the conclusion that "fetal" fibrinogen is less responsive to thrombin, thereby protecting newborns from thromboembolic complications. The physiologic significance of "fetal" fibrinogen is not known.

Thrombin Inhibition: Thrombin activity is regulated by several mechanisms. The 3 plasma inhibitors of thrombin are antithrombin III (ATIII), heparin cofactor II (HCII) and $\alpha_2$macroglobulin (α_2M). At birth and during the first weeks of life, plasma concentrations of ATIII and HCII are approximately 50% of adult values.[26-28,34-47] One anticipates that inhibition of thrombin will be reduced in infants, placing them at risk for thrombotic complications. The rate of inhibition of thrombin is slower in newborn plasmas, but the total capacity is similar to adult plasmas due to increased complex formation with α_2M.[5,48] In contrast to ATIII and HCII, newborn plasma concentrations of α_2M are increased over adult values at birth and are approximately twice adult values by 6 months of age.[4,49] The increased plasma concentrations of α_2M compensate, in large part, for the low plasma concentrations of ATIII (Fig. 2).

In addition to the increased binding of thrombin to α_2M in newborn plasma, there is a small but significant increase in the amount of thrombin bound to HCII. The latter reflects a circulating dermatan sulfate proteoglycan that catalyzes thrombin inhibition by the natural inhibitor HCII.[50] This fetal anticoagulant has properties similar to the dermatan sulfate (DSPG)[50-52], present in plasmas from pregnant women. The length of time that the DSPG remains in newborn blood is not known, except that it is still present during the first week of life in sick infants with respiratory distress syndrome.[48]

The plasma concentrations of ATIII increase to adult values by approximately 3 months of age. In contrast, plasma concentrations of α_2M values remain increased until the third decade of life.[4,49] *In vitro*, plasmas from children inhibit more thrombin than plasmas from adults due to increased binding to α_2M.[25] The increased plasma concentrations of α_2M during childhood probably contribute to the lower risk of thrombotic events in children, including children with congenital heterozygote ATIII deficiency.[6] In the presence of therapeutic concentrations of heparin, thrombin is inhibited to the same extent in plasmas from infants, children and adults. Further, ATIII is the inhibitor responsible for over 95% of the complex formation.

When thrombin is generated *in vivo*, it binds to the endothelial cell surface receptor thrombomodulin (TM). Thrombin bound to TM no longer functions as a coagulant but activates the protein C/protein S

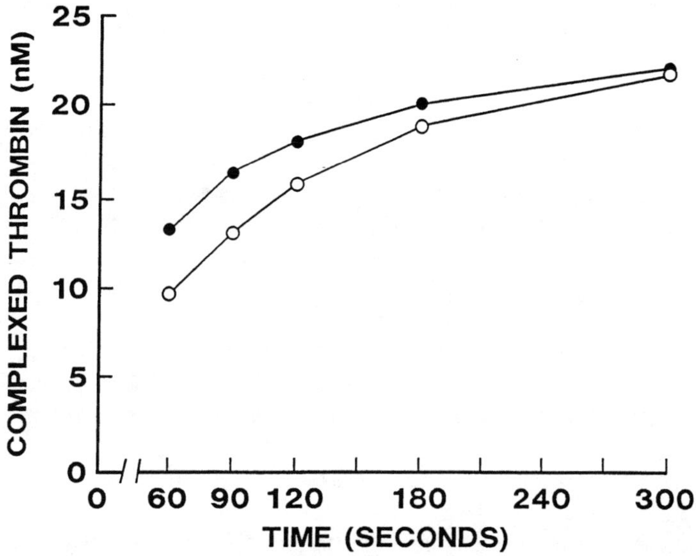

Figure 2. This figure shows that the rate of thrombin inhibition is slower in plasmas from newborns compared to adults. However, the total amount of thrombin inhibited is similar in both plasma systems. Adult ●—●; Newborn ○—○.

inhibitory system by limited proteolysis of protein C to activated protein C (APC). APC inactivates Factors Va and VIIIa by enzymatic degradation. Protein S circulates in plasma in both a free form (active) and complexed with C_4B binding protein.[53,54] At birth, total protein S levels are very low, however, the available protein S is all in the free or active form thereby compensating, at least in part, for the absence of C_4B binding protein.[54] Whether a fetal form of protein S exists is not known at this time. The lower boundary of normal for free protein S is similar throughout childhood to adult values.[4]

Plasma protein C levels are significantly lower in newborns than adults and protein C is present in a fetal form[55], with the two chain form of protein C being twofold higher than in adult plasma. However, there is no evidence at this time that the fetal form of protein C is non-functional. Throughout most of childhood, plasma concentrations of protein C are significantly decreased compared to adults making this an unlikely protective mechanism.[4]

Endogenous Generation of Thrombin: Endogenous activation of coagulation can be quantitated by activation peptides such as prothrombin fragment 1 + 2 (F1 + 2), FPA, and protein C activation peptide; or enzyme-inhibitor complexes such as thrombin-ATIII (TAT), thrombin-α_2M, activated protein C-protein C inhibitor (PCI), and protein C-α_1 anti-trypsin (α_1AT). There is considerable evidence that blood coagulation is activated at the time of birth. Plasma concentrations of FPA, TAT and thrombin-α_2M complexes are increased at birth.[5,56-58] However, this process seems to be well controlled, and self limited. Indeed, activation of coagulation during the birth process does not result in significant consumption of circulating plasma coagulation proteins or clinical morbidity.[59,60] Plasma concentrations of F1 + 2 and TAT are similar in children to young adults (ages 20 to 40 yrs).[4] However, with increasing age (over 40), plasma concentrations of F1 + 2 increase.[61] Further, the thrombin generated is able to act on its natural substrates, fibrinogen and protein C, resulting in age-dependent increases for plasma concentrations of FPA and protein C activation peptide.[61] This *ex vivo* evidence of impaired thrombin regulation in older adults, in combination with *in vitro* evidence of enhanced regulation of thrombin during childhood, together strongly suggest that the regulation of thrombin deteriorates with age, paralleling an increased risk of thrombotic complications.

In summary, there are several mechanisms in place that enhance thrombin regulation during infancy and childhood. These mechanisms may be contributing to the reduced risk of thromboembolic complications. Further, differences in thrombin regulation in plasma from children significantly affect their response to heparin.

B. FIBRINOLYSIS

Once a fibrin clot has formed *in vivo*, the fibrinolytic system lyses the clot to limit its growth. An increased capacity to generate plasmin or a decreased capacity to inhibit plasmin could provide protection from thromboembolic events.

Plasmin Regulation: Both the rate of plasmin generation in plasma[62] and thrombolysis of preformed fibrin clots *in vitro* are impaired significantly in a newborn system compared to the adult.[63] The responsible mechanism for the impaired fibrinolytic response is, at least in part, decreased plasma concentrations of plasminogen (50% of adult) in the presence of nearly adult levels of α_2AP (80% of adult).[1,2,29,34,62-69] In addition, plasminogen is present in a "fetal" form at birth.[70,71] However, the contribution of "fetal" plasminogen to impaired fibrinolysis is unknown.

The capacity of the fibrinolytic system to respond in later childhood has also been assessed and is decreased compared to adults, but by a different mechanism than for newborns.[72] Increased plasma levels of plasminogen activator inhibitor (PAI-1) and decreased plasma concentrations of tissue plasminogen activator (tPA) result in a tPA/PAI-1 ratio that is significantly decreased during childhood (0.37) compared with adults (1.36).[4,72]

In summary, there is no evidence that the fibrinolytic system provides additional protection from thromboembolic complications in childhood. However, a low plasminogen concentration limits the response to thrombolytic agents.[63]

C. THE PLATELET/VESSEL WALL INTERACTION

In addition to the plasma components of hemostasis, the vessel wall provides an important antithrombotic surface under physiologic circumstances. Although not well studied, it is apparent that the vessel wall undergoes an aging process that likely begins in early life. For example, concentrations of vessel wall glycosaminoglycans vary with age[73] and plasma concentrations of the endothelial cell surface receptor, thrombomodulin, are increased at birth and during early childhood.[74] Finally, the bleeding time measurement, which is the only currently available test of platelet vessel interaction *in vivo*, is prolonged during childhood for reasons that are not apparent at this time.[4,75]

D. SUMMARY

In summary, there are several mechanisms in place to protect children from thromboembolic complications. Future research, particularly on the aging of the vessel wall, may uncover other important protective mechanisms. Despite these powerful mechanisms, some children do develop DVT and PE. The subsequent section provides a summary of the epidemiology and treatment of DVT and PE in children.

IV. THE EPIDEMIOLOGY OF DVT/PE IN CHILDREN

Because of the frequency and importance of DVT and PE, these thrombotic complications have been extensively studied in adults. Initial reports on the epidemiology of DVT/PE provided the basis for subsequent, highly successful prophylactic and therapeutic trials.[9,76] In contrast to adults, DVT and PE in children are relatively rare events for which a paucity of information has been available. Two sources of information on the epidemiology of DVT/PE in children have been used for the subsequent section: a comprehensive re-view of the literature[7] and a population-based registry.[14] From 1975 to 1991, 308 children were reported in the English and French literature, with DVT of the extremities and/or PE.[7] The Canadian Registry reported on 137 consecutive children with DVT/PE.[14] The information from these sources is presented under the headings: clinical presentation, diagnostic evaluation, therapeutic interventions and clinical outcome.

A. CLINICAL PRESENTATION

Age Distribution: The age distribution of children with DVT/PE is shown in Figure 3.[7,14] Children less than 1 year of age and teenagers are at greatest risk for DVT/PE. If one includes newborns[8], then the first year of life is clearly the time of greatest risk for DVT/PE in children. The incidence appears to increase during adolescence, with the slight decrease in late teen years reflecting referral to adult services.[77,78] There is no difference between the sexes.

Underlying Disorders: Idiopathic DVT/PE occurs in less than 5% of children with clots compared to approximately 40% of adults with clots.[7,14] The most common underlying diagnoses include cancer, trauma/surgery and congenital heart disease (Fig. 4). Like adults, inherited prethrombotic disorders are documented in only a minority of children. However, the majority of children are not evaluated for congenital prethrombotic disorders, making it possible that the true incidence will be greater than the reported 6 to 11 %.[7,14] Inherited deficiencies of Protein C, Protein S and ATIII are the most common inherited disorders identified. For the vast majority of children with an inherited prethrombotic disorder, an acquired risk for DVT/PE unmasked the deficiency.[7,14,79,80] Although the short-term management of children with DVT/PE and an inherited prethrombotic disorder is relatively straightforward, the long-term management is uncertain.

The predisposing causes of DVT/PE in children are changing. For example, prior to the early 1970s, ventriculo-atrial shunts, infection and congenital heart disease were the leading causes of thromboembolic complications in children.[7,81-84] Ventriculo-atrial shunts are rarely used now because they caused right atrial thrombi and continuous microembolization to the lung with subsequent pulmonary hypertension.[85] Children with cancer, the largest single group of children with DVT in the recent literature and the Canadian registry, rarely survived prior to the late 1960s, to develop DVT.

Location: In adults, DVT in the upper venous system is extremely rare occurring in less than 2% of patients.[86] In striking contrast, DVT in the upper venous system in children accounts for over one third of DVT (Fig. 5). The reason for the frequency of DVT in the upper venous system is solely the use of central venous catheters (CVLs). The presence of CVL is the single most important predisposing cause of DVT in children in both the literature[7] and in the Canadian Registries of neonatal and pediatric thromboembolic complications.[8,14]

Catheter-Related DVT: CVL-related DVT are discussed separately because of the frequency of this complication in children and its unusual clinical presentation. CVL are usually placed for short-term intensive care, or long-term supportive care for children requiring total

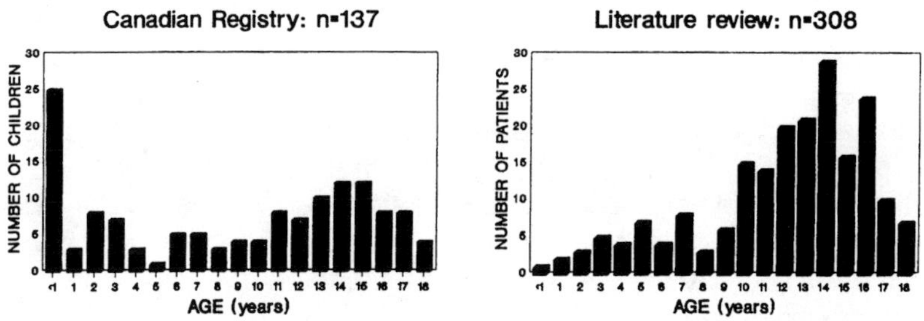

Figure 3. This figure shows the age distribution of children with deep venous thrombosis reported in the literature and in the Canadian registry.

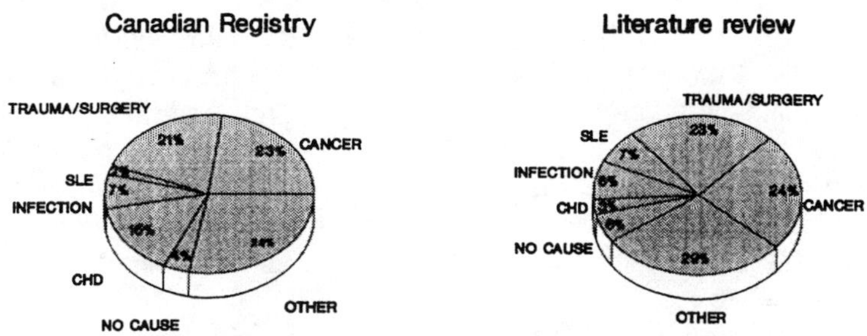

Figure 4. This figure shows the underlying disorders in children with deep venous thrombosis reported in the literature.

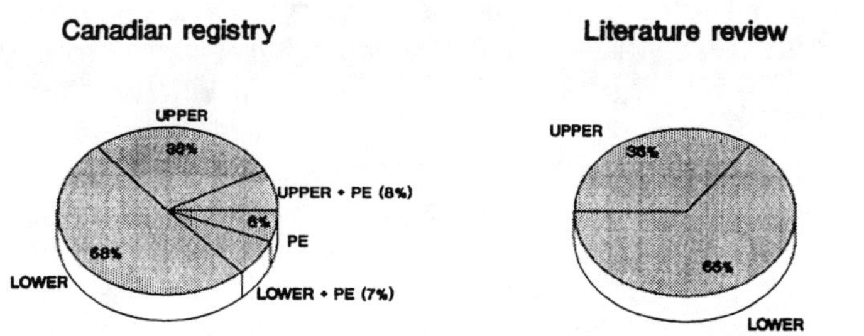

Figure 5. This figure shows the location of DVT in children reported in the literature.

parenteral nutrition (TPN) or therapy for cancer. CVL are thrombogenic because their surfaces are foreign; they damage vessel walls; blood flow is disrupted; and some substances infused are damaging to vessels. Two types of thrombotic complications are described in the literature: fibrin sleeves that are not adherent to vessel walls but may occlude CVL[87], and CVL-related DVT that adhere to vessel walls, partially or completely obstructing vessels around catheters.[87] The occurrence of CVL-related DVT is likely influenced by many parameters such as ratio of CVL to vessel diameter, length of time in place, specific use, and catheter material.

CVL-related DVT can be classified clinically as either asymptomatic or symptomatic. In adult patients, asymptomatic CVL-related DVT is estimated to be 20-fold higher than symptomatic catheter-related DVT.[88,89] The ratio of symptomatic to asymptomatic CVL-related DVT in children is not known. When a CVL "blocks", patency is usually restored with simple measures or local instillation of urokinase.[90-93] If the CVL remains "blocked", it is removed without evaluation with objective tests for DVT. One can argue that this approach is appropriate if there are no clinically important ramifications. However, this is not likely the case. For example, replacement of CVL requires repeated anaesthesia and surgery, with eventual loss of vessel patency in the upper venous system necessitating entry from the lower system. In addition, these children are at risk for clinically symptomatic DVT and/or the long-term complication of postphlebitic syndrome (PPS).

The clinical symptoms of CVL-related DVT, when they occur, include swelling, pain and discoloration of the related limb, swelling of the face, pulmonary embolism (PE)[94], chylothorax[94-97], superior vena cava syndrome[94,95,98-101], and PPS. Symptomatic catheter-related DVT should not be considered benign. Fatal PE do occur secondary to CVL-related DVT, although less frequently than from DVT in the lower limbs.[86,94,101,102] The long-term outcome of CVL-related DVT in children is not known. For adults, only one third to one half of occluded veins recanalize[86,103] and postphlebitic syndrome occurs at least as frequently, if not at a higher rate, than in lower limbs (20-40%).[86,104,105]

In summary, at this time there is no convincing evidence to suggest that CVL-related DVT can be considered benign. The current literature suggests that smaller patients, patients receiving TPN through their CVL[94,106-110] and children requiring hemodialysis[111,112] constitute high risk groups. Effective prophylactic and therapeutic modalities are available if the clinical problem, when more clearly defined, warrants their use.

Non-Catheter-Related DVT and PE: DVT in the lower extremities is the most frequent non-CVL thrombotic complication in children. There have been 203 cases of DVT of the lower extremities and/or PE in children identified in the medical literature, excluding autopsy series (references available on request).[7] The most frequent clinical manifestations of DVT are pain and swelling and redness in the affected extremity. Less frequently there are fever and abdominal or inguinal pain. Asymptomatic DVT has also been discovered during the investigation of PE and postphlebitic syndrome (PPS).[113,114]

The cardinal signs and symptoms of PE in children are also similar to those found in adults. However, there is some evidence for a lower incidence of dyspnea and tachypnea in adolescents or young adults with PE[115], and a higher incidence of signs and symptoms of DVT compared to adult patients.[13] This may reflect both better physiological tolerance in the younger patient and delays in diagnosis.[116,117]

B. DIAGNOSTIC EVALUATION

The diagnosis of DVT in children is complicated by widely diverse locations in which clots occur, small size of the patients, underlying disorders, and lack of validated noninvasive diagnostic radiographic tests. It is well established in adult patients that clinical diagnosis is wrong as often as it is correct. Clinical diagnosis of DVT is likely just as non-specific in children, with only 18% positivity in one retrospective review of venograms performed for clinically suspected DVT.[118] Since 1975, more than 90% of pediatric patients reported have had objective documentation of their diagnosis.

Radiographic Evaluation of DVT: Numerous radiographic techniques are available for the diagnosis of DVT. In general, they can be considered as either invasive (i.e. angiographic study) or non-invasive (i.e. Doppler/ultrasound). In adults, an angiographic study is still considered the reference test against which the sensitivity and specificity of other tests must be compared. Duplex ultrasonography is an attractive alternative to venography for children. However, there are no studies evaluating the sensitivity and specificity of duplex ultrasonography compared to venography in children. Although the positive and negative predictive ability of duplex ultrasonography is excellent for proximal DVT in adults, these results cannot be simply extrapolated to children for many reasons. First, at least one third of DVT in children occur in the upper system where the reliability of duplex ultrasonography has never been compared to venography in well-designed trials. Second, the vessels are usually smaller in children which may pose a further problem. Finally, the effect of the primary disorders, which differ in children from adults, on the reliability of the diagnostic tests is not known. A study to determine the reliability of duplex ultrasonography compared to venography in pediatric patients is urgently needed.

At this time, most thrombotic complications in children should be diagnosed by an angiographic study if possible. For many sick newborns and young infants, transportation to radiology departments is not feasible and bedside ultrasound remains the test of choice. Figure 6 shows the relative proportion of different objective tests used to diagnose both CVL and non-CVL-related DVT in pediatric patients in the literature and in the Canadian Registry.[7,14]

Radiographic Evaluation for Pulmonary Embolism: In reports prior to 1975, PE was usually a surgical or pathological diagnosis. Since 1975, the majority of reported PE in children were diagnosed with lung scan and/or angiography (20% not specified).[7] However, details of lung scan patterns are often missing and ventilation scans were not always performed. In the Canadian Registry, PE was diagnosed in 22 of 31 children based upon high probability VQ scans, for an incidence of 0.86 per 10,000 admissions. This incidence is slightly lower than that previously estimated in adolescents (7.8 per 10,000)[13] and significantly lower than for hospitalized adults.[119] However, only 23% of children were evaluated by VQ scan for PE. The true incidence of PE is likely greater than that documented in the registry reflecting the low index of suspicion of PE in pediatric patients. At this time it is recommended that a ventilation/perfusion scan be performed to investigate suspected PE in pediatric patients.

Catheter-Related DVT: The detection of CVL-related DVT is highly dependent upon the diagnostic test used to investigate a CVL that is "blocked". For example, the frequency of symptomatic occlusion ranges from 1% to 80% in the literature.[91,107,120-129] The lowest frequencies are reported from studies using clinical symptoms of superior vena cava obstruction as evidence for CVL-related DVT and the highest frequencies when venography is used.[107,126] Venography (dye injected into a vein in the hand or foot) should not be confused with injection of dye into CVLs (lineograms). Lineograms are useful for delineating CVL tip location and a clot at the tip of the CVL but cannot be relied upon to detect significant DVT along the intravascular length of the CVL.

C. THERAPEUTIC INTERVENTIONS

The available data clearly support the view that DVT/PE in children requires anticoagulant therapy.[7,14] Recommendations established in adult patients have been extrapolated to children for at least two reasons. First, the incidence of DVT/PE in children is so low that expensive multi-centre trials are required to answer relatively simple dose-related questions. Second, children with DVT/PE present

DIAGNOSIS OF DVT IN CHILDREN

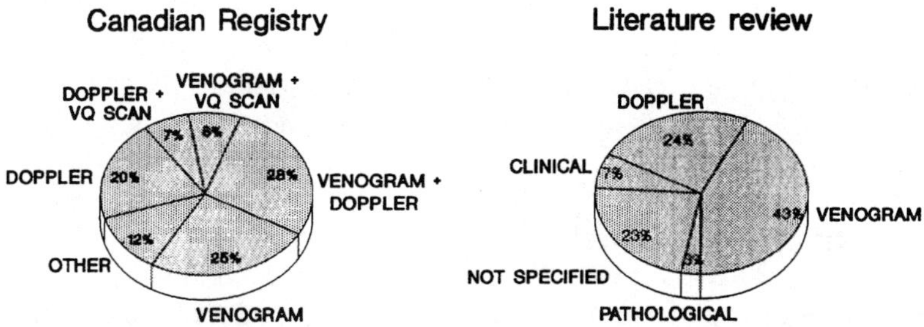

Figure 6. This figure shows the investigations used to diagnose DVT and/or PE.

significant management dilemmas that require immediate therapeutic intervention. Although recommendations for treatment of DVT/PE in adults have been invaluable to children, there are significant limitations (as discussed previously) that necessitate intervention trials in children to determine optimal therapy. The following section provides guidelines for prevention and treatment of DVT/PE in children based upon current recommendations for treatment of DVT/PE in adults and the available information in children.

Heparin Therapy — General: Heparin is the most commonly used anticoagulant in children, for both prophylactic and therapeutic treatment. Heparin is a heterogeneous mixture of polysaccaride chains with molecular chains ranging from 3,000 to 30,000 (mean 15,000). The activities of heparin can be considered as antithrombotic (the ability to prevent thrombosis and to prevent extension of DVT and occurrence of PE) and anticoagulant (the ability to inhibit coagulation enzymes). Heparin mediates these activities by binding to the natural inhibitor ATIII, accelerating the inhibition by ATIII of several coagulation enzymes.[130-133]

The therapeutic range for heparin reflects a minimum adequate level to prevent extension or reoccurrence of DVT/PE and a maximum level to decrease the risk of bleeding.[9,134,135] In hopes of maximizing efficacy and minimizing risks, heparin is monitored by a variety of coagulation tests that provide a measure of the anticoagulant effect of heparin. Although the aPTT is widely used to monitor heparin, the differing sensitivities of aPTT reagents to heparin adversely affects the reliability of the aPTT.[136] To circumvent this problem, currently it is recommended that the therapeutic ranges for aPTT reagents should be standardized to reflect heparin levels of 0.2 to 0.4 by protamine sulphate titration or 0.35 to 0.70 by the anti-Factor Xa assay.[9,137,138] Using an aPTT of 1.5 to 2 times the baseline value without this standardization can no longer be considered adequate monitoring for patients. If the baseline aPTT is prolonged (as in the presence of a non-specific inhibitor) or short (as in the presence of high Factor VIII levels), the aPTT values may not reflect the heparin therapeutic range. When possible, at least one simultaneous aPTT and heparin level should be measured for a patient to ensure that the aPTT reflects the heparin level in that patient. When aPTT values and heparin levels are discordant, heparin levels should be used preferentially because they are a better predictor of the *in vivo* antithrombotic effectiveness of heparin than the aPTT.[139,140] Bleeding complications were rare using this approach.

Recommendations for Treatment of DVT/PE in Adults: Treatment strategies for thromboembolic complications in adults are highly relevant to children. DVT is treated aggressively in adult patients to prevent PE with the potential of sudden death, local extension or reoccurrence, and PPS. Therapy is usually initiated with heparin followed by 3 months of oral anticoagulant therapy.[9] Thrombolytic therapy is controversial, as the evidence of additional benefits are still not clear.[141-143]

The antithrombotic efficacy of heparin in adult patients has been established in randomized, controlled trials that showed both a reduced mortality from PE[144] and a reduced risk of recurrent DVT.[145,146] In addition, achieving therapeutic levels of heparin within 24 hours of initiating therapy reduces the rate of recurrence.[147-151] Informal audits of heparin therapy in adult patients have shown that dose-adjustment practices are often inadequate, delaying the achievement of an aPTT value above the minimum therapeutic level.[152-154] When adult patients are monitored closely with a nomogram, aPTT values above the minimal level are achieved in 82% of patients after 24 hours and in 91% of patients after 48 hours.[154] Current recommendations for adult patients are an initial bolus of 5,000 units/ml of heparin followed by a continuous infusion for an average amount of 30,000 units/24 hours.[9,147,155,156] The duration of heparin therapy can be safely reduced to 4 to 5 days except for patients with massive proximal DVT or pulmonary embolism.[155,156]

Treatment of DVT/PE in Children: In general, DVT/PE are treated with heparin therapy followed by warfarin therapy. Thrombolytic therapy is rarely used (see subsequent section). The general approach to anticoagulant therapy in children has been to achieve adult therapeutic ranges and to treat for similar lengths of time. Unfortunately, dosing of heparin and warfarin in clinical trials in adults have not been reported by body weight so approximations have been used for children. This is important because there is evidence from *in vitro* studies and *in vivo* studies in animals that the activities and pharmacokinetics of anticoagulant and thrombolytic agents may differ in children from adults.[23,62,63,157-160] Recent studies have evaluated protocols for the administration of heparin and warfarin to children and provided information on the doses of these anticoagulants required to achieve adult therapeutic ranges.[161,162] Not surprisingly, there is a significant effect of age.

Heparin Therapy — Children: Therapy with heparin is the most common form of initial treatment for DVT/PE in children as reported in the literature (Fig. 7, see next page). The Canadian Registry provides information on the diversity of clinical practice. Heparin therapy is usually initiated with a bolus of 50 to 100 units/kg, followed by a maintenance dose of 20 to 24 units/kg/hour. The length of therapy varies considerably from 1 to 62 days (median = 14). A recent cohort study formally evaluated a single heparin protocol at one institution in consecutive children with DVT/PE.[162] Therapy was initiated with 50 units/kg as a bolus, followed by an initial maintenance dose of 20 units/kg/hour and adjusted by a heparin nomogram adapted from one used in adults.[154,162] The aPTT was chosen to monitor heparin because the aPTT is inexpensive, widely available and usually reflects heparin concentrations in adult patients. The activated clotting time (ACT), although widely available, was not chosen because it is not as reproducible as the aPTT, is highly operator dependent and significantly influenced by the machine chosen.[163-165] Heparin assays, although better predictors of *in vivo* anti-thrombotic effect, are expensive, and not available on a routine basis. A heparin assay was measured on each patient to confirm that the aPTT was reflecting the heparin concentration. The aPTT therapeutic range recommended for adult patients with DVT was used in the cohort study because it reflected current practice and there was no published alternative.

The results of this study provide basic information on heparin therapy in children.[162] First, a bolus dose of 50 units/kg resulted in only one third of children achieving a therapeutic range 4 hours later. This poor response provides the rationale for giving a larger initial bolus dose of heparin. Second, the amount of heparin/kg/hour varied inversely with age. Plausible explanations for the high heparin requirement in young children are that heparin is cleared more quickly in the young compared to the adult[157,160,166] and/or the delay in diagnosis of DVT in children results in more extensive disease at the time of presentation which may accelerate the clearance of heparin.[167,168] Third, recurrent thrombotic disease, not bleeding, was

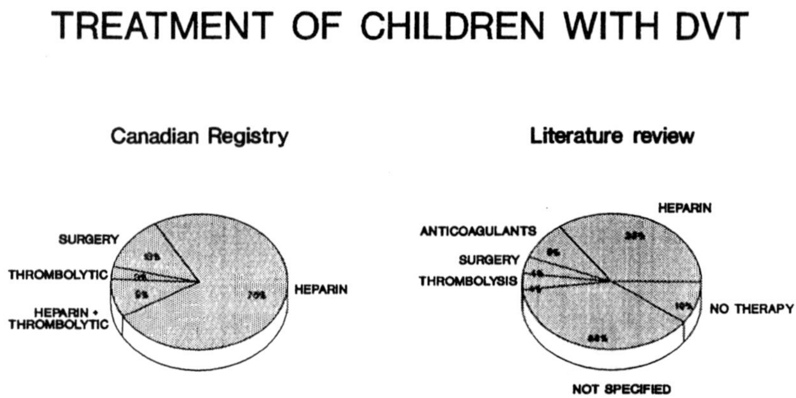

Figure 7. This figure shows the treatments used to manage DVT and/or PE in children.

the clinical complication of concern. Inadequate initial therapy with heparin results in an increased risk of recurrent thrombotic disease in adults.[147-150] Fourth, the aPTT reflected the heparin concentration in approximately 75% of measurements made in children.

Recommendations for Heparin Therapy In Children: Table 1 provides a dosing schedule and a nomogram, based upon aPTT results, for adjusting heparin therapy in children. A bolus dose of 75 to 100 units/kg given over 10 minutes should be followed by a maintenance dose based upon age. Maintenance heparin therapy in infants can be initiated at 28 units/kg/hour and for older children at 20 units/kg/hour. It is important that adjustments are made rapidly to achieve the therapeutic range as soon as possible.[147-150] Except in cases of extensive thrombosis or pulmonary embolism, a short 5 to 7 day course of heparin is likely sufficient and warfarin can be instituted within 48 hours of starting heparin therapy.[155,156] If the aPTT does not prolong appropriately in the presence of average amounts of heparin, it is useful to preferentially adjust the heparin infusion according to the heparin level. One approach is to measure at least one heparin level when the aPTT is therapeutic to ensure that the aPTT reflects the heparin concentration in an individual pediatric patient.

Oral Anticoagulant Therapy — General: Warfarin (4-hydroxy-coumarin) is the oral anticoagulant used most commonly in children. It functions by interfering with vitamin K metabolism. Vitamin K is an essential cofactor for the post-translational carboxylation of glutamic acid (Gla) residues on specific coagulation proteins (protein C, protein S, prothrombin, Factors VII, IX and X). The Gla residues serve as calcium binding sites essential for these coagulation proteins to bind

Table 1
Protocol for Systemic Heparin Administration and Adjustment

1. Loading dose: Heparin 75 units/kg IV over 10 minutes.

2. Intial maintenance dose: 28 units/kg/hour for infants less than 1 year.

3. Intial maintenance dose: 20 units/kg/hour for children over 1 year.

4. Adjust heparin to maintain aPTT 60-85 seconds as follows:

aPTT (SEC)	BOLUS (units/kg) (min)	HOLD CHANGE	%RATE aPTT	REPEAT
< 50	50	0	+10%	4 hrs.
50-59	0	0	+10%	4 hrs.
60-85	0	0	0	next day
86-95	0	0	-10%	4 hrs.
96-120	0	30	-10%	4 hrs.
> 120	0	60	-15%	4 hrs.

5. Obtain blood for aPTT 4 hours after administration of the heparin loading dose and 4 hours after every change in the infusion rate.

6. When aPTT values are therapeutic, a daily CBC, and aPTT.

Abbreviations: Complete blood counts (CBC), activated partial thromboplastin time (aPTT), kilogram (kg), intravenous (IV).

coagulant surfaces for thrombin generation to occur. Warfarin competitively inhibits two enzymes involved in vitamin K metabolism resulting in low plasma concentrations of active forms of these proteins.

The prothrombin time (PT) is sensitive to the reduction of Factors II, VII, and X, and is the most commonly used test for monitoring warfarin therapy.[76,169] Unfortunately, thromboplastin reagents for PT assays have widely varying sensitivities to low plasma concentrations of vitamin K-dependent proteins.[170-174] Prior to recognition of this problem, patients in North America were receiving excessive amounts of warfarin with unnecessary hemo-rrhagic side effects.[175] The international normalized ratio (INR) provides a mechanism of correcting for differing sensitivities of PT reagents.[172-174] The INR is calculated as the patients PT (seconds) divided by the control PT (seconds) to the power of the ISI. The ISI is the international sensitivity index which corrects for the differing sensitivities of various reagents to low levels of the vitamin K-dependent factors. Laboratories involved in monitoring warfarin therapy need to provide INR values to clinicians to facilitate optimal management. The usual therapeutic range for children with DVT/PE is an INR of 2 to 3.

Oral Anticoagulant Therapy — Adults: In adults, heparin therapy is followed by 3 months of oral anticoagulant therapy with warfarin.[76,86,176,177] Current recommendations for adult patients are a loading dose of 10 mg of warfarin for 2 consecutive days followed by the average daily requirement of 4 to 5 mg.[76]

Oral Anticoagulant Therapy — Children: A medline search of the English literature from 1980 to 1993 identified 45 publications describing the use of warfarin in children (references available upon request). More than 80% of reported pediatric patients received warfarin for primary prevention of thromboembolism secondary to prosthetic heart valves, not for secondary prevention of venous thromboembolism. The next largest group identified in the literature was children with homozygous protein C deficiency. There were 2 studies that attempted to determine the epidemiologic features of pediatric patients receiving warfarin.[161,178] One study was a survey based on a questionnaire mailed to 407 haematologists in Great Britain.[178] Based upon a response rate of 58%, the predominant indication for oral anticoagulation was prosthetic cardiac valves (74%). DVT (6%) and inherited prethrombotic disorders (3%) were similarly infrequent.[178] The second study was a prospective cohort study of consecutive patients treated with warfarin at a single institution.[161] The indications for oral anticoagulant therapy in the second study were evenly distributed between secondary prevention of thromboembolism, and primary prevention of systemic thromboembolism in children with congenital heart disease, with or without prosthetic heart valves.

Despite the well-defined need for warfarin in pediatric patients, only a small number of studies were identified that evaluated dose requirements of warfarin in children.[161,179-182] All but one study was conducted prior to the introduction of the INR.[161] The latter study evaluated a single warfarin protocol at one institution in 115 consecutive children.[161] The protocol for warfarin therapy was based upon an earlier study[179] and was initiated with 0.2 mg/kg. Further adjustments were made using a nomogram based upon INR values (Table 2). The length of time required to achieve a minimal INR of 2 ranged from a median of 5 days in patients less than 1 year of age to a median of 3 days in teenagers. The average dose/kg was significantly increased at 0.32 mg/kg in patients less than 1 year of age. The dose requirements gradually decreased with age to 0.09 mg/kg in the older teens. For adults, warfarin dose requirements/kg are not precisely known but are in the range of 0.04 to 0.08 mg/kg for an INR of 2-3.[76] Thus, the requirements for warfarin are significantly increased throughout childhood compared to adults.

The mechanisms responsible for the age-dependent effect of full dose warfarin therapy are not completely clear. However, the

Table 2
Protocol for Warfarin Therapy to Maintain an INR Between 2 and 3

1.	Loading dose 1: If the baseline INR is 1.0 to 1.3: Load with 0.2 mg/kg orally		
2.	Loading doses 2-7: If the INR is:		
	INR	1.1-1.4	repeat loading dose
	INR	1.5-1.9	50% of loading dose
	INR	2.0-3.0	50% of loading dose
	INR	3.0-4.0	25% of loading dose
	INR	>4.5	hold until INR <4.5 then restart at 50% less than previous dose
3.	Long-term Warfarin dose guidelines: If the INR is:		
	INR	1.1-1.4	increase by 20% of dose
	INR	1.5-1.9	increase by 10% of dose
	INR	20-3.0	no change
	INR	3.1-4.0	decrease by 10% of dose
	INR	4.1-4.5	increase by 20% of dose
	INR	> 4.5	hold dose, check INR daily until INR <4.5, then restart at 20% less than previous dose.

particularly high requirements in infants less than 1 year of age were, in part, due to vitamin K supplementation of enteral nutrient formulas. The degree of vitamin K supplementation varies from 55 to 110 μg/litre in the common enteral nutrient formulas. Another cause of relative resistance to warfarin in a smaller number of patients was poor absorption due to short-bowel syndrome[183] despite removal of vitamin K supplementation of their TPN. Enhanced clearance of warfarin is another potential mechanism responsible for the age-dependent dosage requirements.

The duration of warfarin therapy varied with the underlying disorder. Children with DVT and persistent underlying disorders that precipitated the DVTs (most commonly CVLs), were usually treated with a 3 month course of full dose warfarin (INR of 2-3) followed by a low dose regimen (INR of 1.3-1.8) until the precipitating disorder resolved. In some adult patients, low dose warfarin offers a safe and effective alternative to full dose warfarin.[89,184,185]

Monitoring full dose warfarin therapy in children is often difficult and requires close supervision for several reasons including: serious primary problems that influence the biologic effect and clearance of warfarin, noncompliance in teenagers[186,187], and the use of other drugs either on a long-term basis or intermittently. Finally, young children are a particularly difficult group of patients to anticoagulate.[182,187-190] The reported risk of serious bleeding in children receiving warfarin for prophylaxis for mechanical valves ranges from no events to 7.9/100 patient years.[182,187,189-192] The risk of bleeding in adults treated with warfarin for DVT is approximately

3%[76] and for mechanical valves ranges from 1.6 to 7.9/100 patient years.[193] These data suggest that the risk of bleeding while receiving warfarin therapy is similar in children and adults.

DVT Prophylaxis for Children: DVT prophylaxis is of proven benefit for adult patients at high risk for thrombotic complications with risk reductions of 30 to 40%.[10,11,194,195] Standard heparin, low molecular weight heparin (LMWH) and oral anticoagulants are agents used successfully for DVT prophylaxis in adults. Controlled trials of DVT prophylaxis anticoagulant therapy have not been conducted in pediatric patients except in patients with CVLs because the incidence of post-operative thrombosis in children is very low. In one retrospective study of scoliosis, only 8 cases of clinically suspected and objectively documented thromboses were present in 1,229 patients.[21] An incidence of thrombosis of 3.7% was reported in a prospective study of DVT in 54 children on halo-femoral traction, submitted to venography.[196] Thus, there is no evidence to suggest that DVT prophylaxis is warranted in pediatric patients undergoing surgical procedures that are considered high risk in adults patients.

Currently, most children with a CVL receive prophylaxis with heparin in the form of catheter flushes with heparin containing solutions on a regular basis. For external devices this is usually once or twice daily, and for implantable ports, it is a minimum of once every 4 to 6 weeks. The benefits of heparin prophylaxis for maintaining catheter patency have been tested in clinical trials.[197-199] None of these trials could demonstrate a benefit in the form of prolonged patency from heparin flushing of venous catheters. However, some of the studies were for peripheral catheters[198] and CVL-related DVT was not evaluated by venography. One randomized trial of prophylaxis compared once a week saline with more intensive heparin prophylaxis to maintain catheter patency and showed no difference between the two regimens for CVL-related DVT detected by echocardiography.[199] However, differences from centre to centre for patient population, type of catheter used, duration of catheter use, solutions infused and surgical technique may result in a variable risk of catheter-related thrombosis. At this time, it seems prudent to recommend that heparin prophylaxis continues until further studies clarify high risk and low risk pediatric patient populations for CVL-related DVT. For infants it is important to calculate the amount of heparin that is being bolused into the patient because it is quite possible to transiently heparinize these small patients.

Although some low risk pediatric patients may not require heparin prophylaxis in the future, other high risk patients develop CVL-related DVT despite heparin prophylaxis. Infants and children requiring TPN appear to be two groups of pediatric patients at particularly high risk.

Unfortunately, these same children often require further CVLs for prolonged periods of time. A recent randomized trial, conducted in 82 adult patients at high risk of CVL-related DVT, showed a significant benefit from prophylactic low dose warfarin therapy (1 mg daily).[89] The risk reduction for catheter-related DVT diagnosed by venography was 37.5% to 9.5%.[89] Low dose warfarin therapy has also been demonstrated to provide good prophylaxis from DVT in other high risk disorders in adult patients.[200,201] At this time, there is no clear role for warfarin as initial prophylactic therapy for pediatric patients with CVLs.

Thrombolytic Therapy — Children: Thrombolytic therapy is commonly used in low doses, usually to re-establish catheter patency or in systemic doses in children with extensive DVT or massive PE. Streptokinase (SK) should not be used to re-establish catheter patency because of the possibility of allergic reactions with repeated doses. For catheter patency, one commonly used protocol is to instill 2 to 3 ml of Urokinase (UK) (5000 units/ml) for 2 to 4 hours.[90-93] Short infusions of low dose UK have also been used if direct instillation of UK did not re-establish patency. One approach is to infuse UK at 150 units/kg/hour for 8 hours and re-assess with objective tests. Monitoring is advised to ensure that the thrombolytic agent is having an effect. Commonly used tests for monitoring are the fibrinogen concentration, thrombin clotting time, fibrinogen/fibrin degradation products and/or euglobulin lysis time. Systemic dose thrombolytic therapy may be helpful for treatment of massive pulmonary embolism PE, PE not responding to heparin, and for some children with acute, extensive DVT. At this time, the risk/benefit of thrombolytic therapy in children is not known and a general recommendation for thrombolytic therapy cannot be made.

V. CLINICAL OUTCOME

Complications from DVT/PE and its management include recurrent DVT/PE, PPS, bleeding from anticoagulant therapy and death.

Recurrent DVT/PE: In adult patients, the rate of recurrence after DVT is 4 to 7%.[147,155,156] In the Canadian Registry, 124 children survived their primary illness and thrombotic complication. However, recurrent DVT/PE was seen in 23 (18.5%) of children. Children of all ages and with diverse underlying primary problems were affected. Ten of the 23 children had recurrent CVL-related DVT and 4 were Protein C deficient. The recurrent disease was either local in the upper or lower system, or in the form of new PE. Based upon the experience in adults, one can speculate that the high rate of recurrent DVT/PE in children reflects inadequate anticoagulant therapy.

Postphlebitic Syndrome (PPS): The second local complication of DVT is PPS. The symptoms of PPS include swelling, pain, pigmentation, induration of the skin, and ulceration.[202] Symptoms may occur early, or be delayed as long as 5 to 10 years after the initial thrombotic event. PPS is caused by incompetent perforating valves and blood flow directed from the deep system into the superficial system leading to edema and impaired viability of subcutaneous tissues. Only one case series study of PPS in children is identified in the literature. This is a retrospective study in an orthopedic setting.[114] PPS occurred in 8 of 33 (25%) children, a rate comparable to that in adults. The Canadian Registry has identified 26 children (21%) with PPS with a minimum follow up of 6 months.[14] Seven of the children with PPS also had recurrent thromboembolic disease. Further prospective studies are needed to identify the incidence and predisposing features for PPS. Physiologically, it is feasible that the incidence of PPS in children will exceed adults because of the relatively suppressed fibrinolytic system in the young.[4,72]

Bleeding Complications: In contrast to the frequency of recurrent DVT/PE and PPS, bleeding complications secondary to anticoagulant therapy are rarely reported. There are no cases of significant bleeding in children entered in the Canadian Registry.

Mortality: With a follow-up of 18 months, 13 of the 137 children (9.5%) in the Canadian Registry died; 10 from their underlying disease and 3 (2.2%) as a direct result of their thrombotic complications. Two children died of PE, one while receiving anticoagulant therapy, and one was diagnosed at autopsy. In both cases the PE were from CVL-related DVT. The third child died of a thrombus extending into the inferior vena cava while receiving heparin therapy.

VI. CONCLUSIONS

Because of the relatively low incidence of DVT and PE in children, the diagnostic and therapeutic approaches used have been extrapolated from guidelines for adults. This review has shown that the epidemiology of DVT/PE in children differs significantly from adults. Features which differ include: the underlying disorders, the high incidence of CVL-related DVT in the upper venous system, and the response to heparin, warfarin and thrombolytic agents. There is a paucity of information on the risk/benefit ratio of therapeutic interventions and long-term outcome. Clinical trials are needed to clarify optimal management for pediatric patients with DVT/PE.

REFERENCES

1. **Andrew, M., Paes, B., Milner, R., Johnston, M., Mitchell, L., Tollefsen, D.M., Powers, P.** Development of the human coagulation system in the full-term infant. *Blood* 70, 165, 1987.
2. **Andrew, M., Paes, B., Milner, R., Johnston, M., Mitchell, L., Tollefsen, D.M., Castle, V., Powers, P.** Development of the human coagulation system in the healthy premature infant. *Blood* 72, 1651, 1988.
3. **Andrew, M., Schmidt, B., Mitchell, L., Paes, B., Ofosu, F.** Thrombin generation in newborn plasma is critically dependent on the concentration of prothrombin. *Thromb Haemost* 63, 27, 1990.
4. **Andrew, M., Vegh, P., Johnston, M., Bowker, J., Ofosu, F., Mitchell, L.** Maturation of the hemostatic system during childhood. *Blood* 80, 1998, 1992.
5. **Schmidt, B., Mitchell, L., Ofosu, F., Andrew, M.** Alpha-2-macroglobulin is an important progressive inhibitor of thrombin in neonatal and infant plasma. *Thromb Haemost* 62, 1074, 1989.
6. **Mitchell, L., Piovella, F., Ofosu, F., Andrew, M.** Alpha-2-macroglobulin may provide protection from thromboembolic events in antithrombin III deficient children. *Blood* 78, 2299, 1991.
7. **David, M., Andrew, M.** Venous thromboembolism complications in children: A critical review of the literature. *J Pediatr* 123, 337, 1993.
8. **Schmidt, B., Andrew, A.** A prospective international registry of neonatal thrombotic diseases. *Pediatr Res* 1994 (Abstract).
9. **Hirsh, J.** Heparin. *N Engl J Med* 324, 1565, 1991.
10. **Collins, R., Scrimgeour, A., Yusuf, S., Peto, R.** Reduction in fatal pulmonary embolism and venous thrombosis by perioperative administration of subcutaneous heparin: overview of results of randomized trials in general, orthopedic, and urologic surgery. *N Engl J Med* 318, 1162, 1988.
11. **Clagett, G.P., Reisch, J.S.** Prevention of venous thromboembolism in general surgical patients. *Ann Surg* 208, 227, 1988.
12. **Wise, R.C., Todd, J.K.** Spontaneous, lower-extremity venous thrombosis in children. *Am J Dis Child* 126, 766, 1973.
13. **Bernstein, D., Coupey, S., Schonberg, S.K.** Pulmonary embolism in adolescents. *Am J Dis Child* 140, 667, 1986.
14. **Andrew, M., David, M., Adams, M.** Venous thromboembolic complications (VTE) in children: First analyses of the Canadian Registry of VTE. *Blood* 83, 1994.

15. **Coon, W.W., Willis, P.W., Keller, J.B.** Venous thromboembolism and other venous disease in the Tecumseh Community Health Study. *Circ* 48, 839, 1973.
16. **Gjores, J.E.** The incidence of venous thrombosis and its sequelae in certain districts in Sweden. *Acta Chir Scand* 206, 1, 1956.
17. **Carter, C., Gent, M.** The epidemiology of venous thrombosis. In: Hemostasis and Thrombosis. *Basic Principles and Clinical Practice*. Colman, R.W., Hirsh, J., Marder, V.J., Salzman, E.W. (eds), J.B. Lippincott Company, Philadelphia, 1982, pp 805.
18. **Planes, A., Vochelle, N., Mansat, C.** Prevention of deep vein thrombosis after total hip replacement by enoxaparin: one daily injection of 40 mg versus two daily injections of 20 mg. *Thromb Haemost* (Suppl 1), 415, 1987.
19. **Hull, R., Delmore, T., Hirsh, J., Gent, M., Armstrong, P., Lofthouse, R., MacMillan, Blackstone, I., Reid-Davis, Detwiler, R.C.** Effectiveness of an intermittent pulsatile elastic stocking for the prevention of calf and thigh vein thrombosis in patients undergoing elective knee surgery. *Thromb Res* 16, 37, 1979.
20. **Leclerc, J., Desjardins, L., Geerts, W., Jobin, F., Delorme, F., Bourgouin, J.** A randomized trial of enoxaparin for the prevention of deep vein thrombosis after major knee surgery. *Thromb Haemost* 65(Suppl), 753, 1991.
21. **Uden, A.** Thromboembolic complications following scoliosis surgery in Scandinavia. *Acta Orthop Scand* 50, 175, 1979.
22. **Schmidt, B., Ofosu, F.A., Mitchell, L., Brooker, L.A., Andrew, M.** Anticoagulant effects of heparin in neonatal plasma. *Pediatr Res* 25, 405, 1989.
23. **Vieira, A., Ofosu, F., Andrew, M.** Heparin sensitivity and resistance in the neonate: An explanation. *Thromb Res* 63, 85, 1991.
24. **Bussel, J.P., Berkowitz, R.L., McFarland, J.G., Lynch, L., Chitkara, U.** Antenatal treatment of neonatal alloimmune thrombocytopenia. *N Engl J Med* 319, 1374, 1988.
25. **Andrew, M., Mitchell, L., Vegh, P., Ofosu, F.** Thrombin regulation in children differs from adults in the absence and presence of heparin. Submitted to *Thromb Haemost*, 1993.
26. **Hathaway, W., Corrigan, J.** Report of scientific and standardization subcommittee on neonatal hemostasis. *Thromb Haemost* 65, 323, 1991.
27. **Corrigan, J.J.** Normal hemostasis in fetus and newborn. Coagulation. In: Neonatal and fetal medicine. *Physiology and Pathophysiology*. Polin, R.A., Fox, W.W. (eds), Grune and

Stratton, New York, 1991, pp 52.
28. **Hathaway, W.E., Bonnar, J.** Hemostatic disorders of the pregnant woman and newborn infant. Elsevier Science Publishing Co., New York, 1987.
29. **Andrew, M., Paes, B., Johnston, M.** Development of the hemostatic system in the neonate and young infant. *Am J Pediatr Hematol/Oncol* 12, 95, 1990.
30. **Xi, M., Beguin, S., Hemker, H.C.** The relative importance of the factors II, VII, IX and X for the prothrombinase activity in plasma of orally anticoagulated patients. *Thromb Haemost* 62, 788, 1989.
31. **Witt, I., Muller, H., Kunter, L.J.** Evidence for the existence of fetal fibrinogen. *Thromb Diath Haemorrh* 22, 101, 1969.
32. **Hamulyak, K., Nieuwenhuizen, W., Devillee, P.P., Hemker, H.C.** Re-evaluation of some properties of fibrinogen purified from cord blood of normal newborns. *Thromb Res* 32, 301, 1983.
33. **Galanakis, D.K., Mosesson, M.W.** Evaluation of the role of in vivo proteolysis (fibrinogenolysis) in prolonging the thrombin time of human umbilical cord fibrinogen. *Blood* 48, 109, 1976.
34. **Aballi, A.J., de Lamerens, S.** Coagulation changes in the neonatal period and in early infancy. *Pediatr Clin North Am* 9, 785, 1962.
35. **Bleyer, W.A., Hakami, N., Shepard, T.H.** The development of hemostasis in the human fetus and newborn infant. *J Pediatr* 79, 838, 1971.
36. **Hathaway, W.E., Bonnar, J.** Bleeding disorders in the newborn infant. In: Perinatal Coagulation. *Monographs in Neonatology.* Oliver, T.K., Jr. (ed), Grune and Stratton, New York, 1978, pp 115.
37. **Gross, S.J., Stuart, M.J.** Hemostasis in the premature infant. *Clin Perinatol* 4, 259, 1977.
38. **Buchanan, G.R.** Neonatal coagulation: normal physiology and pathophysiology. *Clin Haematol* 1, 85, 1978.
39. **Montgomery, R.R., Marlar, R.A., Gill, J.C.** Newborn haemostasis. *Clin Haematol* 14, 443, 1985.
40. **Gibson, B.** Neonatal haemostasis. *Arch Dis Child* 64, 503, 1989.
41. **Gobel, U., Voss, H.C., Petrich, C., Jurgens, H., Oliver, A.** Etiopathology and classification of acquired coagulation disorders in the newborn infant. *Klin Wochenschr* 57, 81, 1979.
42. **Buchanan, G.R.** Coagulation disorders in the neonate. *Pediatr Clin North Am* 33, 203, 1986.
43. **McDonald, M.M., Hathaway, W.E.** Neonatal haemorrhage and thrombosis. *Semin Perinatol* 7, 213, 1983.

44. **Strothers, J., Boulton, F., Wild, R., Ibbotson, R., Millar, P., Lloyd, M., Snodgrass, H.** Neonatal coagulation (letter). *Lancet* 1, 408, 1975.
45. **Bahakim, H., Gader, A., Galil, A., Babbar, F.A-A., Gaafar, T.H., Edrees, Y.B.** Coagulation parameters in maternal and cord blood at delivery. *Ann Saudi Med* 10, 149, 1990.
46. **Peters, M., Jansen, E., ten Cate, J.W., Kahle, L.H., Ockelford, P., Breederveld, C.** Neonatal antithrombin III. *Br J Haematol* 58, 579, 1984.
47. **Manco-Johnson, M.** Neonatal antithrombin III deficiency. *Am J Med* 87(Suppl 3B), 49S, 1989.
48. **Shah, J.K., Mitchell, L.G., Paes, B., Ofosu, F.A., Schmidt, B., Andrew, M.** Thrombin inhibition is impaired in plasma of sick neonates. *Pediatr Res* 31, 391, 1992.
49. **Ganrot, P.O., Schersten, B.** Serum α_2-macroglobulin concentration and its variation with age and sex. *Clin Chim Acta* 15, 113, 1967.
50. **Andrew, M., Mitchell, L., Paes, B., Berry, L., Burrows, R., Khambalia, B., Ofosu, F.** An anticoagulant dermatan sulphate proteoglycan circulates in the pregnant women and her fetus. *J Clin Invest* 89, 321, 1992.
51. **Muller, A.D., Van Doorm, J.M.** Heparin like inhibitor of blood coagulation in normal newborn. *Nature* 267, 616, 1977.
52. **Matzch, T., Bergqvist, D., Bergqvist, A., Hodson, S., Dawes, J., Hedner, U., Ostergaard, P.** No transplacental passage of standard heparin or an enzymatically depolymerized low molecular weight heparin. *Blood Coag Fibrinol* 2, 273, 1991.
53. **Moalic, P., Gruel, Y., Body, G., Foloppe, P., Dalahousse, B., Leroy, J.** Levels and plasma distribution of free and c_4b-BP-bound Protein S in human fetuses and fullterm newborns. *Thromb Res* 49, 471, 1988.
54. **Schwarz, H.P., Muntean, W., Watzke, H., Richter, B., Griffin, J.H.** Low total protein S antigen but high protein S activity due to decreased c_4b-binding protein in neonates. *Blood* 71, 562, 1988.
55. **Greffe, B.S., Marlar, R.A., Manco-Johnson, M.** Neonatal protein C: Molecular composition and distribution in normal term infants. *Thromb Res* 56, 91, 1989.
56. **Yuen, P.M.P., Yin, J.A., Lao, T.T.H.** Fibrino-peptide A levels in maternal and newborn plasma. *Eur J Obstet Gynecol* 30, 239, 1989.
57. **Suarez, C.R., Gonzalez, J., Menendez, C., Fareed, J., Fresco, R., Walenga, J.** Neonatal and maternal platelets: Activation at time of birth. *Am J Hematol* 29, 18, 1988.

58. **Suarez, C.R., Menendez, C.E., Walenga, J.M., Fareed, J.** Neonatal and maternal hemostasis. Value of molecular markers in the assessment of hemostatic status. *Semin Thromb Haemost* 10, 280, 1984.
59. **Kisker, C.T., Robillard, J.E., Clarke, W.R.** Development of blood coagulation-a fetal lamb model. *Pediatr Res* 15, 1045, 1981.
60. **Andrew, M., O'Brodovich, H., Mitchell, L.** The fetal lamb coagulation system during normal birth. *Am J Hematol* 28, 116, 1988.
61. **Bauer, K.A., Weiss, L.M., Sparrow, D., Vokonas, P.S., Rosenberg, R.D.** Aging-associated changes in indices of thrombin generation and protein C activation in humans. *J Clin Invest* 80, 1527, 1987.
62. **Corrigan, J., Sluth, J.J., Jeter, M., Lox, C.D.** Newborn's fibrinolytic mechanism: Components and plasmin generation. *Am J Hematol* 32, 273, 1989.
63. **Andrew, M., Brooker, L., Paes, B., Weitz, J.** Fibrin clot lysis by thrombolytic agents is impaired in newborns due to a low plasminogen concentration. *Thromb Haemost* 68, 325, 1992.
64. **Corrigan, J.** Neonatal thrombosis and the thrombolytic system. Pathophysiology and therapy. *Am J Pediatr Hematol/Oncol* 10, 83, 1988.
65. **Kolindewala, J.K., Das, B.K., Dube, B., Bhargava, B.** Blood fibrinolytic activity in neonates: Effect of period of gestation, birth weight, anoxia and sepsis. *Ind Pediatr* 24, 1029, 1987.
66. **Runnebaum, I.B., Maurer, S.M., Daly, L., Bonnar, J.** Inhibitors and activators of fibrinolysis during and after childbirth in maternal and cord blood. *J Perinat Med* 17, 113, 1989.
67. **Ambrus, C.M., Jung, O., Ambrus, J.L., Mirand, E.A., Choi, T.S., Bartfay-Szabo, A.** The fibrinolysin system and its relationship to disease in the newborn. *Am J Pediatr Hematol/Oncol* 1, 251, 1979.
68. **Ginsberg, J.S., Hirsh, J., Rainbow, A.J., Coates, G.** Risks to the fetus of radiologic procedures used in the diagnosis of maternal venous thromboembolic disease. *Thromb Haemost* 61, 189, 1989.
69. **Reverdiau-Moalie, P., Gruel, Y., Delahousse, B., Rupin, A., Huart, M., Body, G., Leroy, J.** Comparative study of the fibrinolytic system in human fetuses and in pregnant women. *Thromb Res* 61, 489, 1991.
70. **Edelberg, J.M., Enghild, J.J., Pizzo, S.V., Gonzalez-Gronow, M.** Neonatal plasminogen displays altered cell surface binding and activation kinetics. Correlation with increased glycosylation

of the protein. *J Clin Invest* 86, 107, 1990.

71. **Summaria, L.** Comparison of human normal, full-term, fetal and adult plasminogen by physical and chemical analyses. *Haemost* 19, 266, 1989.
72. **Siegbahn, A., Ruusuvaara, L.** Age dependence of blood fibrinolytic components and the effects of low-dose oral contraceptives on coagulation and fibrinolysis in teenagers. *Thromb Haemost* 60, 361, 1988.
73. **Kumar, V., Berenson, G.S., Ruiz, H., Dalferes, E.R., Strong, J.P.** Acid mucopolysaccharides of human aorta. Part 1. Variations with maturation. *J Atheroscler Res* 7, 573, 1967.
74. **Aurousseau, M.H., Amiral, J., Boffa, M.C.** Level of plasma thrombomodulin in neonates and children. *Thromb Haemost* 65, 1232, 1991 (Abstract).
75. **Sanders, J.M., Holtkamp, C.A., Buchanan, G.R.** The bleeding time may be longer in children than in adults. *Am J Ped Hematol/Oncol* 12, 314, 1990.
76. **Hirsh, J.** Oral anticoagulant drugs. Review article. *N Engl J Med* 324, 1865, 1991.
77. **Robin, M., Boyer, C.** Causes des thromboses veineuses de l'enfant et de l'adolescent en dehors de la periode neonatale. *Arch Fr Pediatr* 44, 467, 1987.
78. **Nguyen, L.T., Laberge, J.M., Guttman, F.M., Albert, D.** Spontaneous deep vein thrombosis in childhood and adolescence. *J Pediatr Surg* 21, 640, 1986.
79. **De Stefano, V., Leone, G., Carolis, M.P., Ferrelli, R., De Carolis, S., Pagano, L., Tortorolo, G., Bizzi, B.** Antithrombin III in fullterm and preterm newborn infants: Three cases of neonatal diagnosis of AT III congenital defect. *Thromb Haemost* 57, 329, 1987.
80. **Mannucci, P.M., Tripodi, A., Bertina, R.M.** Protein S deficiency associated with "juvenile" arterial and venous thromboses. *Thromb Haemost* 55, 440, 1986.
81. **Tyler, H.R., Clark, D.B.** Cerebrovascular accidents in patients with congenital heart disease. *AMA Arch Neurol Psych* 77, 483, 1957.
82. **Jones, D.R.B., Macintyre, I.M.C.** Venous thromboembolism in infancy and childhood. *Arch Dis Child* 50, 153, 1975.
83. **Nachbur, B., Baumgartner, G., Huser, H.J.** Deep thrombophlebitis of the lower extremities in children. *VASA* 53, 1979.
84. **Janin, Y., Becker, J., Wise, L., Schneider, K., Schwartz, D., So, H.** Superior vena cava syndrome in childhood and adolescence: A review of the literature and report of three

cases. *J Pediatr Surg* 17, 290, 1982.

85. **Noonan, J.A., Ehmke, D.A.** Complications of ventriculovenous shunts for control of hydrocephalus. Report of three cases with thromboemboli to the lungs. *N Engl J Med* 269, 70, 1963.
86. **Lindblad, B., Bergqvist, D.** Aggressive or conservative treatment in subclavian vein thrombosis. In: *Controversies in the Management of Venous Disorders*. Eklof, B., Gjores, J.E., Thulesius, O., Bergqvist, D. (eds), Butterworth & Co., London, 1989, pp 141.
87. **Williams, E.C.** Catheter-related thrombosis. *Clin Cardiol* 13, 34, 1990.
88. **Burri, C., Ahnfeld, F.W.** *The Caval Catheter*. Springer-Verlag, Berlin, 1, 1978.
89. **Bern, M.M., Lokich, J.J., Wallach, S.R., Bothe, A., Jr., Benotti, P.N., Arkin, C.F., Greco, F.A., Huberman, M., Moore, C.** Very low doses of warfarin can prevent thrombosis in central venous catheters. A randomized prospective trial. *Ann Intern Med* 112, 423, 1990.
90. **Kellam, B., Fraze, D., Kanarek, K.S.** Clot lysis for thrombosed central venous catheters in pediatric patients. *J Perinatol* 19, 7(3), 242, 1987.
91. **Mirro, J., Jr., Rao, B.N., Stokes, D.C., Austin, B.A., Kumar, M., Dabe, G.V., Colten, M., Balas, L., Rafferty, M., Hancock, M., Fairclough, D.** A prospective study of Hickman/Broviac catheters and implantable ports in pediatric oncology patients. *J Clin Oncol* 7, 214, 1989.
92. **Morris, J.B., Occhionero, M.E., Gauderer, M.W.L., Stern, R.C., Doershuk, C.F.** Totally implantable vascular access devices in cystic fibrosis: A four-year experience with fifty-eight patients. *J Pediatr* 117, 82, 1990.
93. **Winthrop, A.L., Wesson, D.E.** Urokinase in the treatment of occluded central venous catheters in children. *J Pediatr Surg* 19, 536, 1984.
94. **Mollitt, D.L., Golladay, E.S.** Complications of TPN catheter-induced vena caval thrombosis in children less than one year of age. *J Pediatr Surg* 18, 462, 1983.
95. **Le Coultre, C., Oberhansli, I., Mossaz, A., Bugmann, P., Faidutti, B., Belli, D.C.** Postoperative chylothorax in children: differences between vascular and traumatic origin. *J Pediatr Surg* 26, 519, 1991.
96. **Kramer, S.S., Taylor, G.A., Garfinkel, D.J., Simmons, M.A.** Lethal chylothoraces due to superior vena caval thrombosis in infants. *Am J Radiol* 137, 559, 1981.
97. **Dhande, V., Kattwinkel, J., Alford, B.** Recurrent bilateral pleural

effusions secondary to superior vena cava obstruction as a complication of central venous catheterization. *Pediatr* 72, 109, 1983.

98. **Tanaka, K., Takao, M., Yada, I., Yuasa, H., Kusagawa, M., Deguchi, K.** Alterations in coagulation and fibrinolysis associated with cardiopulmonary bypass during open heart surgery. *J Cardiothorac Anesth* 3, 181, 1989.
99. **Graham, L., Jr., Gumbiner, C.H.** Right atrial thrombus and superior vena cava syndrome in a child. *Pediatr* 73, 225, 1984.
100. **Bertrand, M., Presant, C.A., Klein, L., Scott, E.** Iatrogenic superior vena cava syndrome. A new entity. *Cancer* 54, 376, 1984.
101. **Mulvihill, S.J., Fonkalsrud, E.W.** Complications of superior versus inferior vena cava occlusion in infants receiving central total parenteral nutrition. *J Pediatr Surg* 19, 752, 1984.
102. **Rockoff, M.A., Gang, D.L., Vacanti, J.P.** Fatal pulmonary embolism following removal of a central venous catheter. *J Pediatr Surg* 19, 307, 1984.
103. **Swinton, N.W., Jr., Capt., Edgett, J.W., Jr., Major, Hall, R.J., Col.** Primary subclavian-axillary vein thrombosis. *Circ* 38, 737, 1968.
104. **Tilney, N.I., Griffiths, H.J.G., Edwards, E.A.** Natural history of major venous thrombosis of the upper extremity. *Arch Surg* 101, 792, 1970.
105. **Painter, T.D., Karpf, M.** Deep venous thrombosis of the upper extremity, five years experience at a university hospital. *Angiology* 35, 743, 1984.
106. **Ryan, J.A., Jr., Abel, R.M., Abbott, W.M., Hopkins, C.C., Chesney, T. McC., Colley, R., Phillips, K., Fischer, J.E.** Catheter complications in total parenteral nutrition. A prospective study of 200 consecutive patients. *N Engl J Med* 290, 757, 1974.
107. **Marzinotto, V., Adams, M., Pencharz, P., Burrows, P., Andrew, M.** Catheter related thrombosis in children receiving home TPN: Incidence, diagnosis, management. *Thromb Haemost* 69, 1079, 1993 (Abstract).
108. **Wakefield, A., Cohen, Z., Craig, M., Connolley, P., Jeejeebhoy, K.N., Silverman, R., Levy, G.A.** Thrombogenicity of total parenteral nutrition solutions: I. Effect on induction of monocyte/ macrophage procoagulant activity. *Gastroenterology* 97, 1210, 1989.
109. **Wakefield, A., Cohen, Z., Rosenthal, A., Craig, M., Jeejeebhoy, K.N., Gotlieb, A., Levy, G.A.** Thrombogenicity of total parenteral nutrition solutions. II. Effect on induction of

endothelial cell procoagulant activity. *Gastroenterology* 97, 1220, 1989.

110. **Montemurr, P., Lattanzio, A., Chetta, G., Lupo, L., Caputi-Iambrenghi, L., Rubino, M., Giordano, D., Semeraro, N.** Increased in vitro and in vivo generation of procoagulant activity (Tissue Factor) by mononuclear phagocytes after intralipid infusion in rabbits. *Blood* 65, 1391, 1985.
111. **Franzone, A.J., Tucker, B.L., Brennan, L.P., Fine, R.N., Stiles, Q.R.** Hemodialysis in children. *Arch Surg* 102, 592, 1971.
112. **Idriss, F.S., Nikaidok, L.R., King, R., Swenson, O.** Arteriovenous shunts for hemodialysis in infants and children. *J Pediatr Surg* 6, 639, 1971.
113. **Marcinski, A., Barral, V., Sauvegrain, J.** Acquired deep venous thrombosis in children. *Pediatr Radiol* 15, 300, 1985.
114. **Norotte, G., Glorion, C., Rigault, P., Merckx, J., Padovani, J.P., Finidori, D., Bernieve, M.** Complications thromboemboliques en orthopedie pediatrique. Recueil "multicentrique" de 33 observations. *Chir Pediatr* 30, 193, 1989.
115. **Green, R.M., Meyer, T.J., Dunn, M., Glassroth, J.** Pulmonary embolism in younger adults. *Chest* 101, 1507, 1992.
116. **Carson, J.L., Kelley, M.A., Duff, A., Weg, J.G., Fulkerson, W.J., Palevsky, H.I., Schwartz, J.S., Thompson, B.T., Popovich, J.J.R., Hobbins, T.E., Spera, M.A., Alavi, A., Terrin, M.L.** The clinical course of pulmonary embolism. *N Engl J Med* 326, 1240, 1992.
117. **Buck, J.R., Connors, R.H., Coon, W.W., Weintraub, W.H., Wesley, J.R., Coran, A.G.** Pulmonary embolism in children. *J Pediatr Surg* 16, 385, 1981.
118. **Perlmutt, L., Fellows, K.E.** Lower extremity deep vein thrombosis in children. *Pediatr Radiol* 13, 266, 1983.
119. **Stevenson, G.F., Stevenson, F.L.** Pulmonary embolism in childhood. *J Pediatr* 34, 62, 1949.
120. **Stockwell, M., Adams, M., Andrew, M., Cameron, G., Pai, M., Barr, R.** Central venous catheters in children with malignant disorders. *Arch Dis Child* 58, 633, 1983.
121. **Pegelow, C.H., Narvaez, M., Toledano, S.R., Davis, J., Olticica, C., Buckner, D.** Experience with a totally implantable venous device in children. *AJDC* 140, 69, 1986.
122. **Shulman, R.J., Rahman, S., Mahoney, D., Pokorny, W.J., Bloss, R.** A totally implanted venous access system used in pediatric patients with cancer. *J Clin Oncol* 5, 137, 1987.
123. **Bagnall, H.A., Gomperts, E., Atkinson, J.B.** Continuous infusion of low-dose urokinase in the treatment of central venous

catheter thrombosis in infants and children. *Pediatrics* 83, 963, 1989.

124. **Harvey, W.H., Pick, T.E., Reed, K., Solenberger, R.I.** A prospective evaluation on the Port-a-cath implantable venous access system in chronically ill adults and children. *Surg Gynecol Obstet* 169, 495, 1989.
125. **Hockenberry, M.J., Schultz, W.H., Bennett, B., Bryant, R., Falletta, J.M.** Experience with minimal complications in implanted catheters in children. *Am J Pediatr Hematol/Oncol* 11, 295, 1989.
126. **Moore, R.A., McNicholas, K.W., Naidech, H., Flicker, S., Gallagher, J.D.** Clinically silent venous thrombosis following internal and external jugular central venous cannulation in pediatric cardiac patients. *Anesthesiology* 62, 640, 1985.
127. **Poole, M.A., Ross, M.N., Haase, G.M., Odom, L.F.** Right atrial catheters in pediatric oncology: a patient/parent questionnaire study. *Am J Pediatr Hematol/Oncol* 13, 152, 1991.
128. **Sadiq, H.F., Devaskar, S., Keenan, W.J., Weber, T.R.** Broviac catheterization in low birth weight infants: Incidence and treatment of associated complications. *Crit Care Med* 15, 47, 1987.
129. **Mehta, S., Connors, A.F., Jr., Danish, E.H., Grisoni, E.** Incidence of thrombosis during central venous catheterization of newborns: A prospective study. *J Pediatr Surg* 27, 18, 1992.
130. **Rosenberg, R.D., Lam, L.** Correlation between structure and function of heparin. *Proc Natl Acad Sci USA* 76, 1218, 1979.
131. **Lindahl, U., Backstrom, G., Hook, M., Thunberg, L., Fransson, L-A., Linker, A.** Structure of the antithrombin-binding site of heparin. *Proc Natl Acad Sci USA* 76, 3198, 1979.
132. **Casu, B., Oreste, P., Torri, G.** The structure of heparin oligosaccharide fragments with high anti-(factor Xa) activity containing the minimal antithrombin III-binding sequence. *Biochem J* 197, 599, 1981.
133. **Choay, J., Lormeau, J.C., Petitou, M., Sinay, P., Fareed, J.** Structural studies on a biologically active hexasaccharide obtained from heparin. *Ann NY Acad Sci* 370, 644, 1981.
134. **Levine, M.N., Hirsh, J.** Hemorrhagic complications of anticoagulant therapy. *Semin Thromb Haemost* 12, 39, 1986.
135. **Nieuwenhuis, H.K., Albada, J., Banga, J.D., Sixma, J.J.** Identification of risk factors for bleeding during treatment of acute venous thromboembolism with heparin or low molecular weight heparin. *Blood* 78, 2337, 1991.
136. **Shojania, A.M., Tetreault, J., Turnbull, G.** The variations between heparin sensitivity of different lots of activated partial

thromboplastin time reagent produced by the same manufacturer. *Am J Clin Pathol* 89, 19, 1988.

137. **Refn, I., Vestergaard, L.** The titration of heparin with protamine. *Scand J Clin Lab Invest* 6, 284, 1954.
138. **Teien, A.N., Lie, M.** Evaluation of amidolytic heparin assay method. Increased sensitivity by adding purified antithrombin III. *Thromb Res* 10, 399, 1977.
139. **Chiu, H.M., Hirsh, J., Yung, W.L., Regoeczi, E., Gent, M.** Relationship between the anticoagulant and antithrombotic effects of heparin in experimental venous thrombosis. *Blood* 49, 171, 1977.
140. **Levine, M., Hirsh, J., Gent, M., Turpie, A.G.G., Cruickshank, M., Anderson, D.R., Johnston, M.** A randomized trial comparing the activated thromboplastin time with the heparin assay to monitor heparin therapy in patients with acute venous thromboembolism requiring large daily doses of heparin. *Arch Intern Med* 1994, In press.
141. **Trubestein, G.** Can thrombolytics prevent post-phlebitic syndrome and thromboembolic disease? *Haemostasis* 3, 38, 1986.
142. **Kakkar, V.V., Lawrence, D.** Hemodynamic and clinical assessment after therapy for acute venous thrombosis. A prospective study. *Am J Surg* 54, 1985.
143. **Arnesen, M., Horseth, A., Ly, B.** Streptokinase or heparin in the treatment of deep vein thrombosis. *Acta Med Scand* 211, 65, 1982.
144. **Barritt, D.W., Jordon, S.C.** Anticoagulant drugs in the treatment of pulmonary embolism: a controlled trial. *Lancet* 1, 1309, 1960.
145. **Hull, R., Delmore, T., Genton, E.** Warfarin sodium versus low-dose heparin in the long-term treatment of venous thrombosis. *N Engl J Med* 301, 855, 1979.
146. **Lagerstedt, C.J., Olsson, C-G., Fagher, B.O., Oqvist, B.O., Albrechtsson, U.** Need for long-term anticoagulant treatment in symptomatic calf-vein thrombosis. *Lancet* 2, 515, 1985.
147. **Hull, R.D., Raskob, G., Hirsh, J., Jay, R.M., Leclerc, J.R., Geertz, W., Rosenbloom, D., Sackett, D.L., Anderson, C., Harrison, L., Gent, M.** Continuous intravenous heparin compared to intermittent subcutaneous heparin in the initial treatment of proximal vein thrombosis. *N Engl J Med* 315, 1109, 1986.
148. **Basu, D., Gallus, A., Hirsh, J., Cade, J.** A prospective study of the value of monitoring heparin treatment with the activated partial thromboplastin time. *N Engl J Med* 287, 324, 1972.

149. **Turpie, A.G.G., Robinson, J.G., Doyle, D.J.** Comparison of high-dose with low-dose subcutaneous heparin to prevent left ventricular mural thrombosis in patients with acute transmural anterior myocardial infarction. *N Engl J Med* 320, 352, 1989.
150. **Kaplan, K., Davison, R., Parker, M., Mayberry, B., Feiereisel, P., Salinger, M.** Role of heparin after intravenous thrombolytic therapy for acute myocardial infarction. *Am J Cardiol* 59, 241, 1987.
151. **Camilleri, J.F., Bonnet, J.L., Bouvier, J.L.** Thrombolyse intraveineuse dan l'infarctus du myocarde: influence de la qualite de l'anticoagulation sur le taux de recidives precoces d'angor ou d'infarctus. *Arch Mal Coeur* 81, 1037, 1988.
152. **Wheeler, A.P., Jaquiss, R.D., Newman, J.H.** Physician practices in the treatment of pulmonary embolism and deep vein thrombosis. *Arch Intern Med* 148, 1321, 1988.
153. **Fennerty, A., Thomas, P., Backhouse, G., Bentley, P., Campbell, I.A., Routledge, P.A.** Audit of control of heparin treatment. *BMJ* 290, 27, 1985.
154. **Cruickshank, M.K., Levine, M.N., Hirsh, J., Roberts, R., Siguenza, M.** A standard heparin nomogram for the management of heparin therapy. *Arch Intern Med* 151, 333, 1991.
155. **Gallus, A., Jackaman, J., Tillett, J., Mills, W., Wycherley, A.** Safety and efficacy of warfarin started early after submassive venous thrombosis or pulmonary embolism. *Lancet* 2, 1293, 1986.
156. **Hull, R.D., Raskob, G.E., Rosenbloom, D.** Heparin for 5 days as compared with 10 days in the initial treatment of proximal venous thrombosis. *N Engl J Med* 322, 1260, 1990.
157. **Andrew, M., Ofosu, F.A., Schmidt, B., Brooker, L., Hirsh, J., Buchanan, M.R.** Heparin clearance and ex vivo recovery in newborn piglets and adult pigs. *Thromb Res* 52, 517, 1988.
158. **Schmidt, B., Buchanan, M.R., Ofosu, F., Brooker, L., Hirsh, J., Andrew, M.** Antithrombotic properties of heparin in a neonatal piglet model of thrombin induced thrombosis. *Thromb Haemost* 60, 289, 1988.
159. **Schmidt, B., Mitchell, L., Ofosu, F., Andrew, M.** Standard assays underestimate the concentration of heparin in neonatal plasma. *J Lab Clin Med* 112, 641, 1988.
160. **McDonald, M.M., Jacobson, L.J., Hay, W.W., Hathaway, W.E.** Heparin clearance in the newborn. *Pediatr Res* 15, 1015, 1981.
161. **Andrew, M., Marzinotto, V., Brooker, L., Adams, M., Ginsberg, J., Freedom, R., Williams, W.** Oral anticoagulant therapy in

pediatric patients: A prospective study. *Thromb Haemost* 71, 265, 1994.

162. **Andrew, M., Marzinotto, V., Blanchette, V., Ginsberg, J., Burrows, P., Benson, L., Williams, W., David, M., Poon, A., Sparling, C.** Heparin therapy in pediatric patients: A prospective cohort study. *Pediatr Res* 35, 78, 1994.
163. **Green, T.P., Ischam-Schopf, B., Steinhorn, R.H., Smith, C., Irmiter, R.J.** Whole blood activated clotting time in infants during extracorporeal membrane oxygenation. *Crit Care Med* 18, 494, 1990.
164. **Andrew, M., MacIntyre, B., Williams, W.G., Gruenwald, C., Johnston, M., Burrows, F., Wang, E., MacMillan, J., Adams, M.** Heparin therapy during cardiopulmonary bypass requires ongoing quality control. *Thromb Haemost* 70, 937, 1993.
165. **Keeth, J., Trickey, T., King, E., Stafford, T., McInnis, R., Reed, C.** A clinical evaluation of the hemotec ACT. *Proc Am Acad Cardio Perf* 9, 22, 1988.
166. **Turner Gomes, S., Nitschmann, E., Benson, L., Burrows, P., Andrew, M.** Heparin is cleared faster in children with congenital heart disease than adults. *J Am Coll Cardiol* 21, 59a, 1993 (Abstract).
167. **Hirsh, J., van Aken, W.G., Gallus, A.S., Dollery, C.T., Cade, J.F., Yung, W.L.** Heparin kinetics in venous thrombosis and pulmonary embolism. *Circ* 53, 691, 1976.
168. **Chiu, H.M., van Aken, W.G., Hirsh, J., Regoeczi, E., Horner, A.A.** Increased heparin clearance in experimental pulmonary embolism. *J Lab Clin Med* 90, 204, 1977.
169. **Quick, A.J., Grossman, A.M.** Prothrombin concentration in newborns. *Proc Soc Exp Biol Med* 41, 227, 1939.
170. **Loeliger, E.A., van den Besselaar, A.M.H.P., Lewis, S.M.** Reliability and clinical impact of the normalization of the prothrombin times in oral anticoagulant control. *Thromb Haemost* 53, 148, 1985.
171. **Roy, A.J., Jaffe, N., Djerassi, I.** Prophylactic platelet transfusions in children with acute leukemia: A dose response study. *Transfusion* 13, 283, 1973.
172. **Poller, L.** Progress in standardization anticoagulation control. *Hematol Review* 1, 225, 1987.
173. **Poller, L.** Laboratory control of oral anticoagulants. *BMJ* 294, 1184, 1987.
174. **International Committee for Standardization in Haematology, International Committee on Thrombosis and Haemostasis.** ICSH/ICTH Recommendations for reporting prothrombin time in oral anticoagulant control. *Thromb Haemost* 53, 155, 1985.

175. **Hirsh, J., Poller, L., Deykin, D., Levine, M., Dalen, J.E.** Optimal therapeutic range for oral anticoagulants. *Chest* 95, 5S, 1989.
176. **Harley, D.P., White, R.A., Nelson, R.J., Mehringer, C.M.** Pulmonary embolism secondary to venous thrombosis of the arm. *Am J Surg* 147, 221, 1984.
177. **Adams, J.T., McEvoy, R.K., DeWeese, J.A.** Primary deep venous thrombosis of upper extremity. *Arch Surg* 91, 29, 1965.
178. **Evans, D.I.K., Rowlands, M., Poller, L.** Survey of oral anticoagulant treatment in children. *J Clin Pathol* 45, 707, 1992.
179. **Doyle, J.J., Koren, G., Chen, M.Y., Blanchette, V.S.** Anticoagulation with sodium warfarin in children: Effect of a loading regimen. *J Pediatr* 113, 1095, 1988.
180. **Carpentieri, U., Nghiem, Q.X., Harris, L.C.** Clinical experience with an oral anticoagulant in children. *Arch Dis Child* 51, 445, 1976.
181. **Bradley, L.M., Midgley, F.M., Watson, D.C., Getson, P.R., Scott, L.P.** Anticoagulation therapy in children with mechanical prosthetic cardiac valves. *Am J Cardiol* 56, 533, 1985.
182. **Woods, A., Vargas, J., Berri, G., Kreutzer, G., Meschengieser, S., Lazzari, M.A.** Antithrombotic therapy in children and adolescents. *Thromb Res* 42, 289, 1986.
183. **Lehman, M.E., Kolb, K.W., Barnhart, G.R., Wagman, L.D., Barr, W.H.** Warfarin absorption in a patient with short-bowel syndrome. *Clin Pharm* 4, 325, 1985.
184. **Fordyce, M.J., Baker, A.S., Staddon, G.E.** Efficacy of fixed minidose warfarin prophylaxis in total hip replacement. *BMJ* 303, 219, 1991.
185. **Poller, L., McKernan, A., Thomson, J.M., Elstein, M., Hirsch, P.J., Jones, J.B.** Fixed minidose warfarin: a new approach to prophylaxis against venous thrombosis after major surgery. *BMJ* 295, 1309, 1987.
186. **Kumar, S., Haigh, J.R.M., Rhodes, L.E., Peaker, S., Davies, J.A., Roberts, B.E., Feely, M.P.** Poor compliance is a major factor in unstable outpatient control of anticoagulant therapy. *Thromb Haemost* 62, 729, 1989.
187. **Stewart, S., Cianciotta, D., Alexson, C., Manning, J.** The long-term risk of warfarin sodium therapy and the incidence of thromboembolism in children after prosthetic cardiac valves. *J Thorac Cardiovasc Surg* 93, 551, 1987.
188. **McGrath, L.B., Gonzalez-Lavin, L., Edlredge, W.J., Colombi, M., Restrepo, D.** Thromboembolic and other events following valve replacement in a pediatric population treated with antiplatelet agents. *Ann Thorac Surg* 43, 285, 1987.

189. **Spevak, P.J., Freed, M.D., Castaneda, A.R., Norwood, W.I., Pollack, P.** Valve replacement in children less than 5 years of age. *J Am Cardiol* 8, 901, 1986.
190. **Harada, Y., Imai, Y., Kurosawa, H., Ishihara, K., Kawada, M., Fukuchi, S.** Ten-year follow-up after valve replacement with the St. Jude Medical prosthesis in children. *J Thorac Cardiovasc Surg* 100, 175, 1990.
191. **El Makhlouf, A., Friedli, B., Oberhansli, I., Rouge, J.C., Faidutti, B.** Prosthetic heart valve replacement in children. *J Thorac Cardiovasc Surg* 93, 80, 1987.
192. **Rao, S., Solymar, L., Mardini, M.K., Fawzy, M.E., Guinn, G.** Anticoagulant therapy in children with prosthetic valves. *Ann Thorac Surg* 47, 589, 1989.
193. **Stein, P.D., Alpert, J.S., Copeland, J., Dalen, J.E., Goldman, S., Turpie, A.G.G.** Antithrombotic therapy in patients with mechanical and biological prosthetic heart valves. *Chest* 102, 445S, 1992.
194. **Kakkar, V.V., Corrigan, T.P., Fossard, D.P.** Prevention of fatal postoperative pulmonary embolism by low doses of heparin. *Lancet* 2, 45, 1975.
195. **Layvraz, P.F., Richard, J., Bachmann, F., VanMelle, G., Treyraud, J.M., Livio, J.J., Candartjis, G.** Adjusted versus fixed-dose subcutaneous heparin in the prevention of deep-vein thrombosis after total hip replacement. *N Engl J Med* 300, 954, 1983.
196. **Leslie, I.J., Dorgan, J.C., Bentley, G.** Deep venous thrombosis in child during halo-femoral traction. *Lancet* ii, 847, 1979.
197. **Gillies, H., Rogers, H.J., Johnston, J., Harper, P.G., Rudge, C.J.** Is repeated flushing of Hickman catheters necessary? *BMJ* 290, 1708, 1985.
198. **Lombardi, T.P., Gundersen, B., Zammett, L.O., Walters, J.K., Morris, B.** Efficacy of 0.9% sodium chloride injection with or without heparin sodium for maintaining patency of intravenous catheters in children. *Clin Pharm* 7, 832, 1988.
199. **Smith, S.M., Dawson, S.M., Hennessey, R., Andrew, M.** Maintenance of the patency of indwelling central venous catheters: Is heparin necessary. *Am J Pediatr Hematol/Oncol* 13, 141, 1991.
200. **Powers, P.J., Gent, M., Jay, R.M., Julian, D.H., Turpie, A.G.G., Levine, M., Hirsh, J.** A randomized trial of less intense postoperative warfarin or aspirin therapy in the prevention of venous thromboembolism after surgery for fractured hip. *Arch Intern Med* 149, 771, 1989.

201. **Francis, C.W., Marder, V.J., Evarts, C.M., Yaukookbodi, S.** Two-step warfarin therapy: prevention of postoperative venous thrombosis without excessive bleeding. *JAMA* 249, 374, 1983.

202. **Lensing, A.W.A., Hirsh, J., Buller, H.R.** Diagnosis of venous thrombosis. In: Hemostasis and Thrombosis. *Basic Principles and Clinical Practice*. Colman, R.W., Hirsh, J., Marder, V.J., Salzman, E.W. (eds), J.B. Lippincott Company, Philadelphia, 1994, pp 1316.

Chapter 8

THE ROLE OF THROMBIN INHIBITION IN THROMBOLYTIC THERAPY

Martin Prins, Bruno Girolami and Enrico Bernardi

I. INTRODUCTION

Thrombin plays a pivotal role in clot formation and in addition thrombin is incorporated in the clot, thereby influencing its thrombogenicity. Any clot, whether functional or pathologic, is subjected to endogenous fibrinolysis. Moreover, many pathologic clots that cause acute symptoms are subjected to pharmacologic fibrinolysis. The purpose of this chapter is to examine the role and usefulness of the inhibition of thrombin in conjunction with thrombolytic treatment.

II. THROMBIN FUNCTION IN THROMBOLYSIS

A. THROMBOLYSIS

There is convincing evidence that coronary thrombosis plays a pivotal role in the pathogenesis of acute mycardial infarction.[1-4] Consequently, the use of thrombolytic agents in these patients has been studied extensively. Their use has been demonstrated to be associated with improved early infarct-related vessel patency[5,6], improved regional and global left ventricular function[7,8], and with reduced early and late mortality.[9-12]

However, current regimens of thrombolytic therapy in patients with acute myocardial infarction fail to obtain primary patency of infarct-related coronary arteries in approximately a third of cases.[5-7,13-16] This finding may be of major clinical relevance, since there is strong evidence that patients in whom early patency of the infarct-related vessel is not achieved have a worse prognosis with regard to likelihood of survival, infarct size,[17-19] and residual left ventricular function.[20]

Furthermore, reocclusion after thrombolytic therapy may seriously limit the successful treatment of patients with acute myocardial infarction[21,22], since reocclusion occurs in initially recanalized vessels in as many as 20% of patients[15,21] and is related to reinfarction.[13,22]

B. THE THROMBUS DURING AND AFTER THROMBOLYSIS

1. Thrombin and Early Patency

Coronary occlusion in man is usually initiated by plaque fissuration

0-8493-7649-1/95/$0.00+$.50

which leads to thrombus formation and, according to the size and location of the artery involved, causes various clinical syndromes ranging from angina to myocardial infarction and sudden cardiac death. Atheromatous plaque rupture, and arterial wall injuries, in general, expose tissue factor present in both the arterial wall and the plaque itself.[23-25] Thus, the extrinsic coagulation pathway is initiated and large amounts of thrombin are produced and incorporated in the growing thrombus.[24] Thrombin, in turn, is the most potent known activator of platelets.[25] Morphologic studies revealed that coronary thrombi are rich in platelets at the fissuration site, while being mainly composed of fibrin and erythrocytes at the extremities.[14] Thus, a coronary thrombus is usually referred to as having a "white head" and a "red tail".[14,15] The white platelet-rich thrombi have been shown to be less sensitive to thrombolysis as compared to red thrombi.[15] The distribution of platelets within the thrombus mass might also be important. The relative predominance of platelets at the proximal site, the white head, would represent an almost "impermeable core" to thrombolytic agents alone[14,15], because of the plasminogen activator inhibitors present on the surface of platelets. Thrombolysis may also be influenced by the presence of thrombin on fibrin strands within the clot and thrombin associated with the prothrombinase complex on the platelets surface. It is known that the presence of activated platelets markedly amplifies thrombin formation by the prothrombinase complex[23] and, therefore, is likely to be an important factor in fibrin accretion to an existing thrombus. Consistent with this, patients with acute myocardial infarction are shown to have increased levels of markers of thrombin activity before the institution of any therapy.[26] These biochemical considerations are the basis for thrombin inhibition to improve early patency rates when using thrombolytic drugs.

Further arguments for a potential role of thrombin inhibition in improving early patency is the observation that unfractionated heparin or the low molecular weight heparin (Enoxaparin) does not influence thrombolysis by tissue-type plasminogen activator as previously thought, but rather the apparent enhancement of thrombolysis in the presence of (low molecular weight) heparin is due to diminished clot accretion.[27] Furthermore, soon after initiation of thrombolytic therapy a marked increase in plasma levels of the surrogate markers of thrombin activity (fibrinopeptide A and thrombin-antithrombin III complexes) are observed, which in turn can be curtailed by the administration of a bolus of intravenous heparin.[28]

2. Thrombin and Reocclusion

Increased activation of both thrombin and platelets during and after thrombolysis has been demonstrated[29], and has been implicated not only in delayed or failed recanalization but also in reocclusion after initially successful recanalization. Several different mechanisms have been suggested to account for the persistence of a procoagulant state during and after thrombolytic therapy. The most probable two of these are:

1) the persistent expression of procoagulant factors associated with arterial wall injury.[30,31] This is mainly related to the presence of active tissue factor at relatively high concentrations in the atherosclerotic plaque[31-33], which could lead to activation of both the intrinsic and extrinsic coagulation pathways[34-36]; and

2) the procoagulant effects of the thrombus itself[37-38], linked to fibrin-bound thrombin which remains active within the thrombus mass. Although it is conceivable that the amount of thrombin in a residual thrombus mass is insufficient to account for re-thrombosis, based on the direct action of thrombin on fibrinogen[37-41], it is conceivable that fibrin-bound thrombin is capable of initiating the amplification loops of the coagulation system, thereby augmenting the hypercoagulably state. This may be particularly important in low-flow states. In addition, fibrin-bound thrombin is resistant to inhibition by antithrombin III.[42]

Thus, direct inhibition of thrombin may not only facilitate thrombolysis but also is likely to be the most effective way to prevent recurrent thrombus formation, and therefore, prevent reocclusion.[43,44]

III. THROMBIN INHIBITION IN THROMBOLYSIS

A. ANIMAL STUDIES

In recent years, there have been several studies in dogs, rabbits and rats investigating the effects of the inhibition of thrombin as an adjunct to thrombolytic treatment of an experimental-formed thrombus. The interpretation of the results of these studies has been complicated by differences among species, differences in the thrombosis models that were used, and differences in the dosing schedules and pharmacokinetics of the drugs used. Another complication when summarizing the results of these studies is the large variety of outcome measures reported, e.g. percentage of clot lysis after a certain time, time to clot lysis, incidence of and time to reperfusion, incidence and time of reocclusion, and total time of perfusion during the observation period. These outcome measures are all potentially relevant on the premise that an open vessel is clinically important. However, it is currently unclear which of these outcome measures is clinically most relevant.

In nine of the ten studies identified, recombinant tissue-type plasminogen activator was used to induce thrombolysis, while in

Table 1
Design of Animal Studies that Evaluated the Role of Thrombin Inhibition in Thrombolytic Treatment of Experimental Thrombosis

Reference	Model	Method of damage	Thrombolytic regimen
Haskel 1991	Canine coronary artery	Electrical injury (total=1 mg/kg)	rt-PA[a], 17 µg/kg/min for 60 min
Martin 1992	Canine coronary artery	Electrical injury	unglycosilated rt-PA[a], 0.24 mg/kg bolus
Rudd 1992	Rabbit femoral artery	Artificial arterio-venous shunt	rt-PA[a], 0.1 mg/kg bolus + 0.9 mg/kg/h for 1 h
Yao 1992	Canine coronary artery	Copper coil	rt-PA[a], 40 µg/kg bolus + 4 µg/kg/min
Klement 1992	Rat distal aorta	Balloon damage of endothelium + external constrictor	rt-PA[a], 1 mg/kg bolus + 1 mg/kg for 30 min
Stassen 1993	Canine femoral	Physical trauma + 95% lumen reduction with plastic wire tie	rt-PA[a], 0.05 mg/kg bolus + 0.45mg/kg/h
Lenfors 1993	Rats carotid artery	Focal external heating	rt-PA[a], 100 µg/kg bolus + 8 µg/kg/min
Prager 1993	Canine coronary artery	Electrical injury + artificial stenosis	rt-PA[a], 17 µg/kg/min for 60 min (total=1 mg/kg)
Martin 1993	Canine coronary artery	Electrical injury	unglycosilated rt-PA[a], 0.34 mg/kg bolus
Burke 1993	Canine femoral artery	Boiling saline	r-proUK[b], 50,000 U/kg bolus + 50,000 U/kg in 30 min

[a] Recombinant tissue-type plasminogen activator. [b] Recombinant pro-urokinase.

one other study pro-urokinase was used. The animal models of thrombosis that were employed and the fibrinolytic regimen used are summarized in Table 1. In eight of the studies, unfractionated heparin was employed to inhibit thrombin. In six other studies, recombinant hirudin and Enoxaparin were used, and in one study each hirulog, and PPACK were used (some of the studies used more than one active drug).

The results obtained with heparin (in one study low molecular weight heparin) in comparison to saline (or placebo) are summarized in Table 2. It can be seen that in the studies that use the lower doses of

Table 2
Summary of Results of Studies Evaluating the Effect of Thrombin Inhibition by Heparin in Thrombolysis of Experimental Thrombosis

Reference	Heparin Dosage	Outcome	Heparin	Placebo
Haskel	150 U/kg bolus	Incidence of reocclusion	5/6	7/7
1991	+ 50 U/kg/h	Time to reocclusion	37±18	18±15*
Rudd	71 U/kg bolus	Lysis time, 30 min old thrombus	15±3	59±6**
1992	+ 15 U/kg/h	Lysis time, 60 min old thrombus	23±3	72±7**
		Time to reocclusion, 30 min old thrombus	53±5	13±2
		Time to reocclusion, 60 min old thrombus	54±8	13±2**
Klement	40 U/kg bolus	Time to clot lysis	7±2	11±2
1992	+ 40 U/kg/h	Vessel patency (% of time)	75±2	64±8
Lenfors	40 U/kg bolus	Thrombus size (mg)	10±3	5±1
1993	+ 0.47 U/kg/min	Blood flow (ml/min)	54±41	67±45
		Patency	1/7	2/7
		Reocclusion	6/7	5/7
Stassen	6 mg/kg[a,b]	Time to reperfusion	19±5	63±27*
1993		Reperfusion	4/4	2/4
		Total patency time	140±13	9±5**
	2 mg/kg[a]	Time to reperfusion	22±5	63±27[c]*
		Reperfusion	4/4	2/4
		Total patency time	120±24	9±5**
Martin	100 U/kg bolus	Reperfusion	9/10	7/10
1993	+ 100 U/kg/h	Time to reperfusion	24±5	30±5
		Reocclusion	7/9	7/7
		Time to reocclusion	17±8	17±11
	200 U/kg bolus	Reperfusion	6/6	7/10[c]
		Time to reperfusion	17±4	30±5
		Reocclusion	3/6	7/7
		Time to reocclusion	61±21	17±11
Burke	500 U bolus	Clot lysis at 4 hrs (%)	85±5	50±4*
1993	+ 350 U/h	Reperfusion	5/8	0.8**

[a] Only the highest dose of (low molecular weight) heparin is displayed in the table. [b] Enoxaparin was used in this group of animals. [c] The same control group was used for comparison in this study. * $p < 0.05$; ** $p < 0.001$. Time = minutes unless indicated otherwise.

heparin (Rudd et al.[46], Lenfors et al.[50] and Klement et al.[48]) the effect of heparin on the outcome measures (clot lysis, patency and reocclusion) is not very impressive. However, in the studies of Haskel et al.[45], Yao et al.[47], Stassen et al.[49] and Burke et al.[55], that used higher dosages of heparin, impressive, statistically significant differences are observed on clot lysis, time to reperfusion and reocclusion.

The results obtained with hirudin or hirudin fragments[52-54] in comparison to saline (or placebo) are summarized in Table 3. In all but one study, there were favourable trends for hirudin in compar-

Table 3
Summary of Results of Studies Evaluating the Effect of Thrombin Inhibition by Hirudin in Thrombolysis of Experimental Thrombosis

Reference	Hirudin Dosage	Outcome	Hirudin	Placebo
Haskel	1.5 mg/kg bolus	Incidence of reocclusion	0/6	7/7**
1991	+ 1.5 mg/kg/h	Time to reocclusion	-	18±15
Martin	1 mg/kg/h	Total patency time	130±12	48±13
1992		Reperfusion	7/8	4/6
		Coronary Blood Flow (ml/min)	63±2	1±1
Rudd	0.3 mg/kg/h	Half-time for clot lysis	6±1	12±2[c]*
1992				
Klement	1 mg/kg bolus	Time to clot lysis	7±2	11±2
1992	+ 2 mg/kg/h	Vessel patency (% of time)	91±2	64±8*
	0.6 mg/kg +[a]	Time to clot lysis	4±2	11±2*
	+ 2 mg/kg/h	Vessel patency (% of time)	94±1	64±8[b]*
Lenfors	0.9 mg/kg bolus	Thrombus size (mg)	2±1	5±1**
1993	+ 0.06 mg/kg/min (15 min)	Blood flow (ml/min)	191±77	67±45**
	+ 0.03 mg/kg/min (15 min)	Patency	4/5	2/7
		Reocclusion	1/5	5/7
Prager	1.5 mg/kg bolus	Time to reperfusion	23±9	31±4
1993	+ 1.5 mg/kg/h	Time to reocclusion	67±32	63±10
		Reocclusion	4/6	5/6

[a] Hirulog was used in this group of animals. [b] The same control group was used for comparison in this study. [c] This result is significant also versus heparin * $p < 0.05$; ** $p < 0.001$.

ison to saline on the various outcome measures, including earlier patency and less reocclusion. Many of these differences were statistically significant. In the other study, there was only a small trend for hirudin towards earlier reperfusion.

PPACK was evaluated only in single study. In the study of Klement et al.[48] PPACK in a dose of 0.5 mg/kg as a bolus followed by 1.4 mg/kg/hr resulted in a significantly reduced time to clot lysis in comparison to saline (4.2 ± 1.9 versus 10.5 ± 1.6 minutes; $p < 0.05$). There was an increased percentage of total time that the vessel was open during the observation period (94.7 ± 1.0 versus 93.9 ± 7.7%; $p < 0.01$).

Thus, there is ample evidence from animal studies, that inhibition of thrombin (using either an antithrombin III-dependent or antithrombin III-independent thrombin inhibitor) leads to earlier recanalization of the occluded vessel, and delays rethrombosis of the recanalized vessel.

B. CLINICAL STUDIES

1. Patency

Currently, there are results available from four clinical studies that

Table 4
Summary of Results of Studies Evaluating the Value of Thrombin Inhibition as an Adjunct to Thrombolysis on Mortality in Acute Myocardial Infarction

Patency

Reference	**Timing**	**Heparin**		**No Heparin**	
TAMI-3, 1989	90 min	50/63	(79%)	54/68	(79%)
HART, 1990	7-24 h	82/100	(82%)	48/93	(52%)
Bleich, 1990	42-72 h	30/42	(71%)	18/42	(43%)
ECSG, 1992	48-120 h	258/310	(84%)[a]	223/299	(75%)[a]
Aust. HF, 1991[b]	7-10 days	73/101	(72%)	71/95	(75%)[c]

[a] Patients receiving aspirin. [b] All patients received 24 hours of high dose intravenous heparin. [c] Patients receiving aspirin and dipyridamole.

have evaluated the effect of giving heparin in conjunction with recombinant tissue-type plasminogen activator on patency of the infarct-related vessel in patients with acute myocardial infarction. In one other study, all patients received recombinant tissue-type plasminogen activator in conjunction with intravenous heparin. Patients were then randomized after 24 hours to either continuation of the intravenous heparin treatment or discontinuation of the heparin and initiation of treatment with aspirin and dipyridamole. The results of these studies are summarized in Table 4. Clinical studies with the newer thrombin inhibitors as an adjunct to thrombolysis have not yet been reported. In the trials using heparin, patency was assessed by angiography which was performed at different times (varying from 90 minutes to 11 days) after the initiation of thrombolytic treatment.

In the third Thrombolysis and Angioplasty in Myocardial Infarction trial [TAMI-3][55] patients with acute myocardial infarction who presented within 6 hours of the onset of symptoms were included. All patients received recombinant tissue-type plasminogen activator (1.5 mg/Kg) over a period of 4 hours (1.0 mg/h over the first hour with 10% given as a bolus; 0.5 mg/h over the following 3 hours). Patients were randomized to receive 10,000 units of heparin intravenously as a bolus (at the start of the infusion of rtPA) or no heparin. Since angiography was performed 90 minutes after initiation of treatment, this dose of heparin is likely to give therapeutic heparin levels for the period until the performance of the angiography. However, this dosage of heparin did not appear to improve the patency at 90 minutes. In the heparin group, 50 out of 63 patients (79%) had a patent infarct-related vessel (TIMI grade 2 and 3), while in the control group, 54 out of 68 (79%) had a patent infarct-related vessel. The 95% confidence interval of this result (-14.8 to 14.8%) implies that it is unlikely that a true benefit of heparin at 90 minutes will be more than 15%.

In the Heparin-Aspirin Reperfusion Trial [HART][56], patients with acute myocardial infarction who presented within 6 hours of the onset of symptoms were included. All patients received a bolus of recombinant tissue-type plasminogen activator (6 mg) followed by a 6 hour infusion (54 mg in the first hour, 20 mg in the second hour and 5 mg over each of the subsequent 4 hours). Patients were randomized to receive either low dose aspirin (80 mg) daily for 7 days, or intravenous heparin (5,000 as a bolus, followed by 1,000 U/hour, adjusted on the basis of the aPTT and continued for 7 days). Coronary angiography was performed at 7 to 24 hours, as well as at day 7 after the start of treatment. The patency (TIMI grade 2 or 3) at 7 to 24 hours was better in patients receiving heparin (82/100, 82%) than in patients receiving aspirin (48/93, 52%). This absolute difference (30%) was statistically significant ($p < 0.001$; 95% confidence interval 16.3 to 41.9%). A repeat coronary angiography was performed on day 7 in those patients who had a successful recanalization as assessed on the first angiogram. Patency was maintained in approximately 90% of the patients, regardless of treatment group. These data indicate that the benefit gained in patency at 7 to 24 hours by adding heparin to thrombolytic treatment is not likely to be decreased by the occurrence of reocclusion of the infarct related vessel within 7 days.

Bleich et al.[57] studied the role of heparin as an adjunct to thrombolytic treatment in patients with acute myocardial infarction who presented within 6 hours after onset of symptoms. All patients received a bolus of recombinant tissue-type plasminogen activator (6 mg over 2 minutes, followed by a 3 hour infusion; 54 mg infused over the first hour, 40 mg over the following 2 hours). Patients were randomized to receive intravenous heparin (5,000 U as a bolus, followed by 1,000 U/hour, adjusted on the basis of the aPTT until the time of angiography) or no heparin. Coronary angiography was performed on day 3 (48-72 hours) after the start of treatment. Patency (TIMI grade 2 or 3) was better in those patients receiving heparin (30/42, 71%) than in those patients receiving rtPA alone (18/42, 43%). This difference (28%) was statistically significant ($p < 0.02$; 95% confidence interval, 5.1 to 49%).

In the European Study Group trial[58], the thrombolytic therapy was started within 6 hours after onset of acute myocardial infarction. All patients received recombinant tissue-type plasminogen activator (10 mg as a bolus, followed by a 3-hour infusion; 50 mg over the first hour; 40 mg over the two subsequent hours) and aspirin (250 mg intravenously or 300 mg orally as a loading dose, followed by 75-125 mg on alternate days). Patients were randomized to receive immediately before the start of recombinant tissue-type plasminogen activator infusion, intravenous heparin (5,000 as a bolus, followed by 1,000 U/hour) or a dilute albumin solution as placebo. The heparin dosage in this study was not adjusted on the basis of the aPTT, and continued at 1,000 U/hour until the time of angiography. Coronary angiography was performed 48-120 hours after the start of treatment. Patency (TIMI grade 2 or 3) was slightly better in those patients receiving heparin (258/310, 83%) than in those patients receiving placebo (223/299, 75%). This difference (8%) was statistically significant ($p < 0.02$; 95% confidence interval, 2.2 to 15.1%).

In the Australian Heart Foundation trial[59], the thrombolytic therapy was started in patients admitted to the hospital within 4 hours of onset of symptoms. All patients received recombinant tissue-type plasminogen activator (10 mg as a bolus, followed by 50 mg infused in the first hour, and 40 mg over the subsequent 2 hours) and heparin for 24 hours (5,000 U as a bolus at the start of the rtPA infusion, followed by an infusion of 1,000 U/hour). Patients were then randomized to receive heparin intravenously (adjusted on the basis of the aPTT) for 7-10 days, or aspirin (300 mg/daily) plus dipyridamole (100 mg t.i.d.). Coronary angiography was performed 7-10 days after randomization (8-11 days after the initiation of thrombolytic treatment). Patency (TIMI grade 2 or 3) was similar among the two groups: 71 out of 95 (75%) in those patients receiving heparin and 73 out of 101 (72%) receiving thrombolytic therapy alone. This difference (3%) was not statistically significant ($p > 0.2$; 95% confidence interval, 10 to 15%).

Finally, one other study enables us to compare the relative effects of intermediate dose subcutaneous heparin (12,500 U, given twice daily) and high dose intravenous heparin (5,000 bolus, followed by 1,000/hour, adjusted on the basis of the aPTT) in patients receiving streptokinase (1.5 MU over 1 hour) as thrombolytic treatment for myocardial infarction. All patients receiving a recombinant tissue-type plasminogen activator, received high-dose intravenous heparin. Patients were randomly assigned to undergo coronary angiography either at 90 or 180 minutes, at 24 hours or at 5-7 days. The patency rate (TIMI grade 2 or 3) at 90 minutes (54 versus 60%), 180 minutes (73 versus 74%) and 24 hours (77 versus 80%) did not differ substantially between the intermediate and high heparin dose groups. However, the patency at 5 to 7 days after start of treatment in the high dose group was 81/96 (84%) and in the intermediate dose group 67/93 (72%). This difference suggested a trend for a heparin dose-related effect (p = 0.051). A repeat coronary angiography was made on day 5 to 7 in the patients who underwent their first angiographic procedure at 90 minutes and who had a successful recanalization as assessed on this angiogram. Patency was maintained in approximately 95% of the patients, regardless of treatment group.

The results of these six clinical studies indicate that the effect on patency rates at 90 minutes after initiation of thrombolytic treatment by inhibiting thrombin by heparin is less than 15%. There is better evidence that at 24 hours there is a substantially increased patency with high dose heparin in comparison to no heparin in patients treated with recombinant tissue-type plasminogen activator. A heparin dose-related effect at 24 hours on patency was not apparent in the GUSTO trial. However, in that study, the patients received streptokinase, all patients received at least an intermediate dosage of heparin, which might, in combination with the fibrin and fibrinogen degradation products generated by streptokinase treatment, provide substantial inhibition of thrombin. There is good evidence that inhibition of thrombin by high dose heparin in comparison with no heparin on day 3 and day 3, 5, results in higher patency rates. One study showed no difference in patency rates on day 7. However, in that study, all patients received heparin initially. Moreover, the comparison was not made with no heparin but with an active drug regimen, i.e. the aspirin plus dipyridamole, which also may influence patency. In the GUSTO trial, there was a favourable result for high dose heparin in comparison to the intermediate dose regimen in patients receiving streptokinase as the thrombolytic agent when patency was measured at day 7 in a random subset of patients. The contrast with the results of the first day angiography in this study, which did not indicate a better effect of high dose heparin over intermediate dose heparin, might be explained by the absence of thrombin inhibition by fibrin and fibrinogen degradation products in the later days after thrombolytic treatment with streptokinase for the myocardial infarction, or the inability of the intermediate dose heparin alone to generate plasma levels within or above the therapeutic level in a substantial proportion of patients.

2. Mortality

The effect of heparin on mortality as an adjunct to thrombolysis in the treatment of patients with acute myocardial infarction was investigated in four large trials: Studio sulla Calciparina nell'Angina e nella Trombosi Ventricolare e nell'Infarto [SCATI][60]; the International Study Group [ISG][61]; the Third International Study of Infarct Survival [ISIS-3][62]; and the Gruppo Italiano per lo Studio della Sopravvivenza nell'Infarto Miocardico [GISSI-2].[63] In these studies, the mortality rates were analyzed at different time points. Three trials reported the in-hospital mortality. The patients enrolled in the GISSI-2 trial were incorporated within the ISG trial patients group and therefore, will not be considered separately in this section. The 35 day mortality was reported for the GISSI-2 and for the ISIS-3 patients. The mortality reported in these trials is summarized in Table 5 (see next page).

In the SCATI trial[60], patients with acute myocardial infarction who presented within 24 hours of the onset of symptoms were randomized to receive heparin (2,000 U intravenously as a bolus, followed 9 hours later by 12,500 U, given subcutaneously b.i.d.), or no heparin. A subset of patients who were admitted within 6 hours from the onset of symptoms, also received thrombolytic treatment with streptokinase (1.5 MU over 1 hour). In this subset, the in-hospital mortality was 10/218 (4.5%) in the patient group who received heparin versus 19/215 (8.8%) in the patient group who did not receive heparin. This difference (4.3%) was statistically significant ($p < 0.05$; crude 95% confidence interval, 0.5 to 9.0%).

In the ISG trial[61], patients with acute myocardial infarction admitted with a duration of symptoms of less than 6 hours were, both randomly allocated to receive recombinant tissue-type plasminogen activator (100 mg over 3 hours) or streptokinase (1.5 MU over 30-60 min) as well as to subcutaneous heparin (12,500 U b.i.d. started 12 hours after the beginning of thrombolytic therapy) or no heparin in a factorial design. No significant difference in hospital mortality was found between patients receiving heparin or no heparin: 884/10,361 (8.5%) versus 932/10,407 (8.9%), respectively. Interestingly, there was a lower fatality rate [408/5,191 (7.9%) versus 479/5,205 (9.2%)] when heparin was given in combination with added to streptokinase ($p < 0.05$). The opposite was observed when heparin was added to recombinant tissue-type plasminogen activator [476/5,170 (9.2%) versus 453/2,502 (8.7%)], difference not significant. However, within patients treated with recombinant tissue-type plasminogen activator, the difference in mortality between the heparin and no heparin group was based almost exclusively on observation in the first 12 hours when heparin had not yet been started.

In the ISIS-3 study[62], patients entering the hospital up to 24 hours after the onset of suspected acute myocardial infarction, were randomized to recombinant tissue-type plasminogen activator (0.60 MU/kg over 6 hours), streptokinase (1.5 MU over 1 hour), or anisoylated plasminogen-streptokinase activator complex (30 U over 3 minutes). All patients received aspirin (162 mg/day). The patients also were randomized to receive subcutaneous heparin (12,500 U b.i.d. started 4 hours after the beginning of thrombolytic therapy for

Table 5
Summary of Results of Studies Evaluating the Value of Thrombin Inhibition as an Adjunct to Thrombolysis on Mortality in Acute Myocardial Infarction

		Mortality			
Reference	**Timing**	**Heparin**		**No Heparin**	
Streptokinase					
SCATI,1989[a]	in hospital mortality	10/218	(4.5%)	19/215	(8.8%)
ISG,1990	in hospital mortality	408/5,191	(7.9%)	479/5,205	(9.2%)
ISIS-3,1992	mortality on day 35	726/13,780	(10.5%)	729/13,780	(10.6%)
Recombinant Tissue-Type Plasminogen Activator					
ISG,1990	in hospital mortality	176/5,170	(9.2%)	453/5,202	(8.7%)
ISIS-3,1992	mortality on day 35	684/13,746	(10.0%)	734/13,746	(10.7%)
Amisoylated Plasminogen-Streptokinase Activator Complex					
ISIS-3,1992	mortality on day 35	722/13,773	(10.5%)	726/13,773	(10.6%)
All Thrombolytic Agents					
ISG,1990	in hospital mortality	884/10,361	(8.5%)	932/10,407	(8.9%)
GISSI-2,1990	mortality on day 35	968/10,014	(9.3%)	983/10,081	(9.4%)
ISIS-3,1992	in hospital mortality	1,534/20,729	(7.4%)	1,633/20,670	(7.9%)
ISIS-3,1992	mortality on day 35	2,132/20,656	(10.3%)	2,189/20,643	(10.6%)

In all studies, patients received heparin 12,500 U subcutaneously twice daily.[a] In the SCATI study, patients received also an initial intravenous bolus of 2,000 U of heparin. In the ISG, GISSI-2 and ISIS-3 studies all patients received aspirin.

7 days) or no heparin. There was no statistical difference in 35 day mortality between the heparin patient group (2,132/20,656; 10.3%) versus the no heparin patient group (2,189/20,653; 10.6%), independently of the thrombolytic drug regimen used. During the hospital stay (day 0-7), there was a trend towards decreased mortality in the heparin group (1,534/20,656; 7.4%) as compared to the no heparin group (1,633/20,643; 7.9%; p = 0.06).

When the in-hospital mortality of these three trials (SCATI, ISG, ISIS-3) are combined, the use of heparin is associated with a 7% relative risk reduction (p <0.03, 95% confidence interval 1 to 12%).

Combining the results of two trials (GISSI-2 and ISIS-3)[62,63] that reported on 35-day mortality, no significant advantage could be observed with the use of heparin [3,100/31,017 (10%) and 3,172/31,050 (10.2%)] in the heparin group and non-heparin group, respectively). In the GUSTO trial, a comparison between two dosage regimens of heparin was made. Intermediate dose subcutaneous heparin (12,500 U, given twice daily) and high dose intravenous heparin (5,000 bolus, followed by 1,000/hour, adjusted on the basis of the aPTT) were compared in patients receiving streptokinase (1.5 MU over 1 hour) as thrombolytic treatment for myocardial infarction. All patients receiving recombinant tissue-type plasminogen activator received high dose intravenous heparin. The 24-hour mortality rates were 274/9,796 (2.8%) in the intermediate dose group and 300/10,377 (2.9%) in the high dose heparin group. The 30-day mortality rates were 705/9,796 (7.2%) and 767/10,377 (7.4%), respectively. None of these results are significantly different.

In conclusion, the combined results of these large-scale trials suggest that using an intermediate dose of heparin which does not prolong the aPTT to a therapeutic level in the majority of patients is associated with a small, but significant reduction of in-hospital mortality. This benefit is most apparent in patients treated with streptokinase. However, the 35-day mortality in the GISSI-2 and ISIS-3 study does not indicate even a trend towards a favourable effect on mortality with this heparin regimen. In the GUSTO trial[64], there also was no difference in 30-day mortality between patients receiving intermediate or high dose heparin. The 95% confidence interval of the difference at day 30 (minus 0.9 to 0.5%) suggests that it is unlikely that the true benefit on mortality of high dose heparin to intermediate dose heparin will be more than 0.5%. To date, there has been no comparison between high dose heparin and no heparin or intermediate dose heparin in patients given recombinant tissue-type plasminogen activator.

IV. CONCLUSION

The benefit of thrombin inhibition in thrombolysis continues to be a subject of debate among clinicians. Laboratory studies high-lighted the central role of thrombin in thrombogenesis, and also provide a sound biological and pathophysiologic rationale for the use of thrombin inhibitors to improve thrombolytic treatment. Initial trials suggested that there was a benefit of using intermediate dose heparin on in-hospital mortality in patients given streptokinase treatment. Later studies, however, cannot confirm this benefit on mortality on in-hospital or day 35 mortality in patients given recombinant tissue-type plasminogen activator (with intermediate dose heparin), or demonstrate a benefit on 30-35-day mortality in patients treated with streptokinase plus high or intermediate dose heparin.

Animal studies, as well as studies in patients with myocardial infarction show that use of thrombin inhibitors (at a proper dosage) is able to improve outcomes related to the patency of the thrombosed vessels. It should be emphasized that almost all of the reported studies used recombinant tissue-type plasminogen activator rather than streptokinase. In animal studies, two groups of thrombin inhibitors have been studied: antithrombin III-dependent inhibitors such as (low molecular weight) heparin, and antithrombin III-independent inhibitors such as hirudin and derivatives. Both types of inhibitors appear to provide some beneficial effect on patency-related outcomes. However, in human studies thus far only heparin has been evaluated.

V. OUTSTANDING ISSUES

Many questions with regard to the clinical usefulness of thrombin inhibition in thrombolysis remain unanswered. For example, improved patency rates may relate to better in-hospital and 1-month term survival, and heparin administration in high doses may be a means to improve those patency rates at 24 to 120 hours after thrombolysis with recombinant tissue-type plasminogen activator. However, it still remains unclear as to why the 1-month mortality rate is not improved in streptokinase-treated patients also receiving intermediate or high dose heparin. In this regard, a trial comparing the effects on mortality of high dose heparin versus no heparin in patients treated with recombinant tissue-type plasminogen activator may be warranted.

In addition, it is not clear whether different antiplatelet therapy regimens have influenced the outcome measures of some of these trials. Antiplatelet drugs such as aspirin are likely crucial adjuncts to thrombolytic treatment in myocardial infarction.[64] The current approach in association with thrombin inhibition may be the application of high dose heparin in patients treated with recombinant tissue-type plasminogen activator, and no or intermediate dose heparin in patients treated with streptokinase. Forthcoming trials evaluating the effects of low molecular weight heparins or antithrombin III-independent thrombin inhibitors on patency and mortality will be of great interest.

REFERENCES

1. **Bertina, R.M.** Molecular basis of thrombosis. In: Protein C and Related Proteins: *Biochemical and Clinical Aspects*. Bertina, R.M. (ed), Churchill Livingstone, Edinburgh, 1988, pp 1-12.
2. **DeWood, M.A., Spores, J., Nortske, M.D., Mouser, L.T., Burroghs, R., Golden, M.S., Lang H.T.** Prevalence of total coronary occlusion during early hours of transluminal myocardial infarction. *N Engl J Med* 303, 897, 1980.

3. **Falk, E.** Unstable angina with fatal outcome: dynamic coronary thrombosis leading to infarction and/or sudden death: autopsy evidence of recurrent mural thrombosis with periferal embolization culminating in total vascular occlusion. *Circ* 71, 699, 1985.
4. **Davies, M.J., Thomas, T.** The pathophysiological basis and microanatomy of occlusive thrombus formation in human coronary arteries. *Phil Trans R Soc Lond B* 294, 225, 1981.
5. **The TIMI Study Group**. The thrombolysis in myocardial infarction (TIMI) trial. Phase 1 findings. *N Engl J Med* 312, 9932, 1985.
6. **Topol, E.J., Calif, R.M., George, B.S., Kerelakes, D.J., Abbottsmith, C.W., Candela, R.J., Lee, K.J., Pitt, B., Stack, K.S., O'Neill, W.W. and the Thrombolysis and Angioplasty in Myocardial Infarction Study Group**. A randomized controlled trial of immediate versus delayed elective angioplasty after intravenous tissue plasminogen activator in acute myocardial infarction. *N Engl J Med* 317, 581, 1987.
7. **National Heart Foundation of Australia Coronary Thrombolysis Group**. Coronary thrombolysis and myocardial salvage by tissue plasminogen activator given up to four hours after onset of myocardial infarction. *Lancet* 1, 203, 1988.
8. **White, H.D., Norris, R.M., Brown, M.A., Takajama, M., Masiowski, A., Bass, N.M., Ormiston, J.A., Whitlock, T.** Effect of intravenous streptokinase on left ventricular function and early survival after acute myocardial infarction. *N Engl J Med* 317, 850, 1987.
9. **Gruppo Italiano per lo Studio della Sterptokinasi nell' Infarto Miocardico (GISSI).** Long-term effects of intravenous thrombolysis in acute myocardial infarction: final report the GISSI study. *Lancet* 2, 871, 1987.
10. **ISIS-2 (Second International Study of Infarct Survival) Collaborative Group**. Randomised trial of intravenous streptokinase, oral aspirin, both, or neither among 17,187 of suspected acute myocardial infarction: ISIS-2. *Lancet* 2, 349, 1988.
11. **Wilcox, R.G., von der Lippe, G., Olsson, C.G., Jensen, G., Skene, A.M., Hampton, J.R.** Trial of tissue plasminogen activator for mortality reduction in acute myocardial infarction. Anglo-Scandinavian Study of Early Thrombolysis (ASSET). *Lancet* 2, 525, 1988.
12. **AIMS Trial Study Group**. Effect of intravenous APSAC on mortality after acute myocardial infarction: preliminary report of a placebo-controlled clinical trial. *Lancet* 1, 545, 1988.
13. **Lavie, C.J., Gersh, B.J., Chesebro, J.H.** Reprefusion in acute myocardial infarction. *Mayo Clin Proc* 65, 659, 1990.

14. **Collen, D.** Coronary thrombolysis: streptokinase or recombinant tissue-type plasminogen activator. *Ann Intern Med* 112, 529, 1990.
15. **Popma, J.J., Topol, E.J.** Adjuncts to thrombolysis for myocardial reperfusion. *Ann Int Med* 115, 34, 1991.
16. **Ohman, E.M., Califf, R.M.** Thrombolytic therapy; overview of clinical trials. *Cor Art Dis* 1, 23, 1990.
17. **The GUSTO Angiographic Investigators.** The effects of tissue plasminogen activator, streptokinase, or both on coronary patency, ventricular function, and survival after acute myocardial infarction. *N Engl J Med* 329, 1615, 1993.
18. **Simoons, M.L., Serruys, P.W., van den Brand, M., Res, J., Verhaught, F.W.A., Krauss, X.H., Remme, W.J., Bar, F., deZwaan, C., van der Laarse, A., Vermeer, F., Lubsen, J.** Early thrombolysis in acute myocardial infarction: limitation of infarct size and improved survival. *J Am Coll Cardiol* 7, 717, 1986.
19. **Hochman, J.S., Ckoo, H.** Limitation of myocardial infarct expansion by reperfusion independent of myocardial salvage. *Circ* 75, 299, 1987.
20. **Res, J.C., Simoons, M.L., van der Wall, E.E., van Eengle, M.J., Vermeer, F., Verheught, F.W., Wijns, W., Braat, S., Remme, W.J., Serruys, P.W., Roos, J.P.** Long term improvement in global left ventricular function after early thrombolytic treatment in acute myocardial infarction. *Br Heart J* 56, 414, 1986.
21. **Johns, J.A., Gold, J.A., Leinbach, H.K., Yasuda, T., Gimple, L.W., Werner, W., Finkelstein, D., Newell, J., Ziskind, A.A., Collen, D.** Prevention of coronary artery reocclusion and reduction in late coronary artery stenosis after thrombolytic therapy in patients with acute myocardial infarction. *Circ* 78, 546, 1988.
22. **Shaer, D.H., Ross, A.M., Wasserman, A.G..** Reinfarction recurrent angina and occlusion after thrombolytic therapy. *Circ* 76(Suppl II), 57, 1987.
23. **Becker, R.C.** Thrombin antagonists and antiplatelet agents. *Am J Cardiol* 69, 39a, 1992.
24. **Maraganore, J.M.** Thrombin, thrombin inhibitors, and the arterial thrombotic process. *Thromb Haemost* 70, 208, 1993.
25. **Heras, M., Chesebro, J.H., Webster, M.W.I., et al.** Hirudin, heparin and placebo during deep arterial injury in the pig: the *in vivo* role of thrombin in platelet-mediated thrombosis. *Circ* 82, 1476, 1990.
26. **Eisenberg, P.R., Sherman, L.A., Schectman, K., et al.** Fibrinopeptide A: a marker of acute coronary thrombosis. *Circ* 71, 912, 1985.

27. **Agnelli, G., Pascucci, C., Cogmi, B., Nenci, G.G.** Effects of hirudin and heparin on the binding of fibrin to the thrombus in t-PA treated rabbits. *Thromb Haemost* 66, 592, 1991.
28. **Rapold, H.J., Kuemmerli, H., Weiss, M., Baur, H., Haeberill, A.** Monitoring of fibrin generation during thrombolytic therapy of acute myocardial infarction with recombinant tissue-type plasminogen activator. *Circ* 79, 980, 1989.
29. **Rapold, H.J.** Promotion of thrombin activity by simultaneous thrombolytic therapy without simultaneous anticoagulation. *Lancet*, 335, 481, 1990.
30. **Heras, M., Chesebro, J.H., Webster, M.W., Mruk, J.S., Grill, D.E., Penny, W.J., Bowie, E.J., Badimon, L., Fuster, V.** Effects of thrombin inhibition on the development of acute platelet-thrombus deposition during angioplasty in pigs. Heparin versus recombinant hirudin, a specific thrombin inhibitor. *Circ* 79, 657, 1989.
31. **Weiss, H.J., Turitto, V.T., Baumgartner, H.R., Nemerson, Y., Hoffman, T.** Evidence for the presence of tissue factor activity on endothelium. *Blood* 73, 968, 1989.
32. **Drake, T.A., Morrissey, J.H., Edgington, T.S.** Selective cellular expression of tissue factor in human tissues. *Am J Pathol* 134, 1087, 1989.
33. **Wilcox, J.N., Smith, K.M., Schwartz, S.M., Gordon, D.** Localization of tissue factor in the normal vessel wall and in the atherosclerotic plaque. *Proc Natl Acad Sci USA* 86, 2839, 1989.
34. **Eisenberg, P.R., Sherman, L.A., Schectman, K., Perez, J., Sobel, B.E., Jaffe, A.S.** Role of new anticoagulants as adjunctive therapy during thrombolysis. *Am J Cardiol* 67, 19a, 1991.
35. **Bach, R.R.** Initiation of coagulation by tissue factor. *CRC Crit Rev Biochem* 23, 339, 1988.
36. **Osterud, B., Rapaport, S.** Activation of factor IX by the reaction product of tissue factor and factor VII: additional pathway for initating blood coagulation. *Proc Natl Acad Sci USA* 74, 5260, 1977.
37. **Weitz, J.I., Hudoba, M., Massel, D., Maraganore, J., Hirsh, J.** Clot-bound thrombin is protected from inhibition by heparin-antithrombin III but is susceptible to inactivation by antithrombin III-independent inhibitors. *J Clin Invest* 86, 385, 1990.
38. **Francis, C.W., Markham, R.E., Jr., Barlow, G.H., Florack, T.M., Dobrzynski, D.M., Marder, V.J.** Thrombin activity of fibrin thrombi and soluble plasmic derivatives. *J Lab Clin Med* 102, 220, 1983.
39. **Kaminski, M., McDonagh, J.** Studies on the mechanism of thrombin interaction with fibrin. *J Biol Chem* 258, 10530, 1983.

40. **Liu, C.Y., Nossel, H.L., Kaplan, K.** The binding of thrombin by fibrin. *J Biol Chem* 254, 10421, 1979.
41. **Wilner, G.D., Danitz, M.P., Mudd, M.S., Hsieh, K., Fenton, J.W.** Selective immobilization of alfa-thrombin by surface-bound fibrin. *J Lab Clin Med* 97, 403, 1981.
42. **Hogg, P.J., Jackson, C.M.** Fibrin monomer protects thrombin from inactivation by heparin-antithrombin III: implications for heparin efficacy. *Proc Natl Acad Sci USA* 86, 3619, 1989.
43. **Jang, I., Gold, H.K., Leinbach, R.C., McNary, J.E., Fallon, J.T., Collen, D.** Acceleration of reperfusion by combination of rt-PA and a selective thrombin inhibitor, argatroban. *Circ* 80(Suppl) II-217, 1989.
44. **Runge, M.S., Bode, C.** Inhibition of platelets and thrombin: implications for treatment of coronary artery thrombosis. *Z Kardiol* 82(Suppl 2), 82, 1993.
45. **Haskel, E.J., Prager, N.A., Sobel, B.E.** Relative efficacy of antithrombin compared with antiplatelet agents in accelerating coronary thrombolysis and preventing early reocclusion. *Circ* 83, 1048, 1991.
46. **Rudd, M.A., George, D., Johnstone, M.T., Moore, R.T., Collins, L., Rabbani, L.E., Loscalzo, J.** Effect of thrombin inhibition on the dynamics of thrombolysis and on platelet function during thrombolytic therapy. *Circ Res* 70, 829, 1992.
47. **Yao, S.K., McNatt, J., Anderson, H.V.** Thrombin inhibition enhances tissue-type plasminogen activator-induced thrombolysis and delays reocclusion. *Am J Physiol* 262, H374, 1992.
48. **Klement, P., Born, A., Hirsh, J.** The effect of thrombin inhibitors on tissue plasminogen activator induced thrombolysis in a rat model. *Thromb Haemost* 68, 64, 1992.
49. **Stassen, J.M., Rapold, H.J., Vanlinthout, I.** Comparative effects of enoxaparin and heparin on arterial and venous clot lysis with alteplase in dogs. *Thromb Haemost* 69, 454, 1993.
50. **Lenfors, S., Marberg, L., Wikstrom, S., Jonsson, U., Eriksson, A.W., Gustafsson, D.** A new rat model of arterial thrombosis with a platelet-rich head and erythrocyte-rich tail: thrombolysis experiments with specific thrombin inhibition. *Blood Coag Fibrinol* 4, 263, 1993.
51. **Prager, N.A., Torr-Brown, S.R., Sobel, B.E., Abendshein, D.R.** Maintenance of patency after thrombolysis in stenotic coronary arteries requires combined inhibition of thrombin and platelets. *J Am Coll Cardiol* 22, 296, 1993.
52. **Martin, U., Fischer, S., Sponer, G.** Influence of heparin and systemic lysis on coronary blood flow after reperfusion induced by the novel recombinant plasminogen activator BM 06.022 in a

canine model of coronary thrombosis. *J Am Coll Cardiol* 22, 914, 1993.

53. **Burke, S.E., Lubbers, N.L., Nelson, R.A., Henkin, J.** Recombinant pro-urokinase requires heparin for optimal lysis and restoration of blood flow in a canine femoral artery thrombosis model. *Thromb Haemost* 69, 375, 1993.
54. **Martin, U., Sponer, G., Strein, K.** Hirudin and sulotroban improve coronary blood flow after reperfusion induced by the novel recombinant plasminogen activator BM 06.022 in a canine model for coronary artery thrombosis. *Int J Hematol* 56, 143, 1992.
55. **Topol, E.J., George, B.S., Kereiakes, D.J., Stump, D.C., Candela, R.J., Abbottsmith, C.W., Aronson, L., Pickel, A., Boswick, J.M., Lee, K.L., Ellis, S.J., Califf, R.M. and the TAMI Study Group.** Randomized controlled trial of intravenous tissue plasminogen activator and early intravenous heparin in acute myocardial infarction. *Circ* 79, 281, 1989.
56. **Hsia, J., Hamilton, W.P., Kleiman, N., Roberts, R., Chaitman, B.R., Ross, A.M.** Heparin-Aspirin Reperfusion Trial (HART) Investigators. A comparison between heparin and low-dose aspirin as adjunctive therapy with tissue plasminogen activator for acute myocardial infarction. *N Engl J Med* 323, 1433, 1990.
57. **Bleich, S.D., Nichols, T.C., Schumacher, R.R., Cooke, D.H., Tate, D.A., Teichman, S.L.** Effect of heparin on coronary arterial patency after thrombolysis with tissue plasminogen activator in acute myocardial infarction. *Am J Cardiol* 66, 1412, 1990.
58. **deBono, D.P., Simoons, M.L., Tijssen, J., Arnold, A.E., Betriu, A., Burgersdijk, C., Lopez Bescos, L., Mueller, E., Pfisterer, M., Van de Werf, F., et al.** Effect of early intravenous heparin on coronary patency, infarct size, and bleeding complications after alteplase thrombolysis: results of a randomised double blind European Cooperative Study Group trial. *Br Heart J* 67, 122, 1992.
59. **Thompson, P.L., Aylward, P.E., Federman, J., Giles, R.W., Harris, P.J., Hodge, R.L., Nelson, G.I., Thomson, A., Tonkin, A.M., Walsh, W.F.** National Heart Foundation of Australia Coronary Thrombolysis Group. A randomized comparison of intravenous heparin with oral aspirin and dipyridamole 24 hours after recombinant tissue-type plasminogen activator for acute myocardial infarction. *Circ* 83, 1534, 1991.
60. **The SCATI (Studio sulla Calciparina nell'Angina e nella Trombosi Ventricolare nell'Infarto) Group.** Randomised

controlled trial of subcutaneous calcium-heparin in acute myocardial infarction. *Lancet* 2, 182, 1989.

61. **The International Study Group.** In-hospital mortality and clinical course of 20,891 patients with suspected acute myocardial infarction randomised between alteplase and streptokinase with or without heparin. *Lancet* 336, 71, 1990.
62. **ISIS-3: (Third International Study of Infarct Survival) Collaborative Group.** A randomised comparison of streptokinase vs tissue plasminogen activator vs anistreplase and of aspirin plus heparin vs aspirin alone among 41,299 cases of suspected acute myocardial infarction. *Lancet* 339, 753, 1992.
63. **GISSI-2: Gruppo Italiano per lo Studio della Sopravvivenza nell'Infarto Miocardico.** A factorial randomised trial of alteplase versus streptokinase and heparin versus no heparin among 12,490 patients with acute myocardial infarction. *Lancet* 336, 65, 1990.
64. **The GUSTO Investigators.** An international randomized trial comparing four thrombolytic strategies for acute myocardial infarction. *N Engl J Med* 329, 673, 1993.

Chapter 9

THROMBOSIS AND PREGNANCY

Jeffrey S. Ginsberg and Patrick Brill-Edwards

I. INTRODUCTION

Pulmonary embolism (PE) is an important cause of maternal mortality.[1,2] Since PE is a potentially preventable and treatable condition, early and accurate diagnosis and treatment are mandatory. However, extra care must be taken when investigating and treating a pregnant patient with clinically suspected venous thromboembolism (VTE) because of potential adverse effects to the fetus from radiation exposure and anticoagulant therapy. Over the last few years, several studies have provided guidelines for the investigation and management of pregnant patients with suspected and established VTE. In this chapter several of these studies will be reviewed and the guidelines for the rational management of thrombotic complications in pregnant patients will be discussed.

II. HYPERCOAGULABILITY AS A CONSEQUENCE OF PREGNANCY

Several physiological changes such as venous stasis, increased levels of clotting factors, and decreased fibrinolytic activity occur during pregnancy, causing hypercoagulability. Decreases in venous tone and venous flow in the lower extremities also occur during pregnancy, causing venous stasis and increasing the likelihood of venous thrombosis.[3,4] In addition, venous outflow obstruction may occur as a consequence of compression of the inferior vena cava and left iliac vein by the gravid uterus.[5]

Alterations in the levels of procoagulant and anticoagulant factors occur during pregnancy and the puerperium. Fibrinogen, Factors VII, X, VIII:C and VIIIR:Ag increase during pregnancy.[6] As a consequence, the prothrombin time (PT) and activated partial thromboplastin time (aPTT) can shorten.[7] Antithrombin III levels have been reported to be normal[6,8,9] or decreased.[10-12] Protein C levels remain normal[10,12] whereas levels of both total and free protein S decrease during pregnancy.[10,13] Increased thrombin generation and activity (measured as elevated levels of thrombin-antithrombin III complexes and fibrinopeptide A as possible consequences of the increase in some procoagulants) and the decrease in anticoagulants, have been reported to occur during

0-8493-7649-1/95/$0.00+$.50

pregnancy.[10,14] The levels of these coagulation factors normalize by 2 weeks post-partum.[6,15,16]

Reduction in global fibrinolytic activity, measured by a prolongation of the euglobulin lysis time, also has been described during pregnancy.[6,17] Plasminogen levels increase during preg-gnancy[11,17,18] but there are conflicting reports about the levels of tissue plasminogen activator (tPA) activity and antigen.[17,18,19] Plasminogen activator inhibitor 1 (PAI 1) levels increase during pregnancy[17,18], and there is the appearance of a second type of plasminogen activator inhibitor, PAI 2. [The PAI 2 species is unique to pregnancy.[17,18]] PAI 1 levels decrease by 50% 1 hour after delivery and return to normal within 3 to 5 days post-partum[17,18,20] whereas PAI 2 levels are still elevated 3 days post-partum.[18] Fibrin degradation products (FDP) are often detectable during late pregnancy.[17,19,21]

To summarize, most of the coagulant changes that occur during pregnancy cause hypercoagulability. One exception is the production, near term, of dermatan sulfate by the placenta.[22] The appearance of this glycosaminoglycan may provide protection against thrombosis and explain the lack of a preponderance of VTE during the third trimester of pregnancy (see below).

III. EPIDEMIOLOGY OF VENOUS THROMBOSIS DURING PREGNANCY

The true incidences of deep vein thrombosis (DVT) and PE during pregnancy and the post-partum period are unknown. The incidences of DVT and PE diagnosed on clinical grounds have been estimated in published reports, but such estimates are likely to be inaccurate because clinical diagnosis is inaccurate.[23] There are two studies in which venography was systematically performed in pregnant women with clinically suspected DVT.[24,25] In the first study, the monthly rate of DVT was estimated to be 0.01/1000 during pregnancy and 0.61/1000 during the post-partum period.[24] The second study reported a monthly rate of 0.8/1000 during pregnancy.[25] Based on the results of studies to date, it is likely that the incidence of VTE is higher during the post-partum period than ante-partum, but it is unclear whether the incidence of VTE is higher in pregnant women than in non-pregnant women.

In a recent cohort study performed at McMaster University in 60 consecutive women with DVT during pregnancy, we found that 58 of the DVTs had occurred in the left leg and the other 2 were bilateral.[26] The preponderance of left leg DVT is consistent with the results of a previous study[25] and may be explained, in part, during pregnancy by the exaggeration of left common iliac vein compression by the right iliac artery where the vessels cross.[27] Since the procoagulant changes are maximal during the third trimester, it might be expected that the risk of thrombosis is highest during the third trimester. However, in the McMaster study, the distribution of DVT events during the first, second and third trimesters was 24%, 47% and 29%, respectively.[26] In another study of 17 patients with objectively proven DVT during pregnancy, Bergqvist et al.[25] reported a similar distribution for the three trimesters (24%, 44% and 31%, respectively). It is possible that the production of dermatan sulfate by the placenta during the third trimester accounts for the lack of preponderance of DVT during the third trimester and slight preponderance of DVT during the second trimester. However, this hypothesis is unproven.

IV. DIAGNOSIS OF DVT/PE DURING PREGNANCY

Frequently, DVT and PE are both present in the same patient and are different clinical manifestations of one disease.[28] The diagnosis of VTE during pregnancy is difficult because clinical diagnosis is inaccurate[7] and leg pain and swelling are common and usually not caused by DVT. Therefore, as in non-pregnant patients, accurate objective tests must be performed when DVT or PE is suspected. The performance of radiologic procedures during pregnancy is problematic because of the fear of exposing the fetus to radiation. The potential risks associated with radiation exposure of the fetus to 5 rads or less have been reviewed critically.[29] There appears to be a slight increase in subsequent childhood cancer but no increase in clinically significant congenital malformations. This study also provides estimates of the amounts of radiation absorbed by the fetus for the different procedures used to diagnose VTE (Table 1).

V. DIAGNOSIS OF DVT

Accurate objective testing is mandatory in pregnant patients with suspected DVT to confirm the diagnosis of DVT and limit the use of anticoagulant therapy, but not without its inherent risks. The estimation of a pre-test likelihood on the basis of clinical signs, symptoms, and patient risk factors is useful when interpreted in conjunction with the results of a non-invasive test. For example, the combination of a high pre-test likelihood and normal impedance plethysmography (IPG) at presentation is associated with a post-test likelihood of DVT of over 50%.[30] Therefore, further investigation (with duplex ultrasonography or venography) is indicated in such

Table 1
Estimated Fetal Radiation With Procedures Used to Diagnose DVT

Procedure (rads)	Estimated Fetal Radiation
Bilateral Venography without abdominal shield	0.628
Unilateral Venography without abdominal shield	0.314
Limited Venography abdomen shielded	<0.050
Pulmonary Angiography via femoral route	0.405
Pulmonary Angiography via brachial route	<0.050
Perfusion Lung Scan using ^{99m}TcMAA	
3 mCi	0.018
1-2 mCi	0.006-0.012
Ventilation Lung Scan:	
using 1^{33}Xe	0.004-0.019
using ^{99m}TC DtPA	0.007-0.035
using ^{99m}TC SC	0.001-0.005
Radioisotope Venography	0.205
Radioactive Fibrinogen Uptake Scanning	2.000
Chest X-Ray	<0.001

Reproduced with permission from Thromb Haemost 1989;61:189-196.

patients.

In non-pregnant patients with DVT, approximately 80% of the thrombioccur in the proximal (popliteal or more proximal) veins, with or without calf DVT, whereas the remaining 20% occur in the calf veins.[31] Approximately 30% of the patients with isolated calf vein thrombosis, develop clinically important extension into the proximal veins within 7 to 14 days of presentation. The remaining 70% of thrombi do not extend and do not require treatment.[31] An approach to the diagnosis of DVT that has been validated in large clinical trials is the performance of a test which is sensitive to proximal DVT, such as IPG or compression ultrasonography

(CUS).[32-35] If the initial test is normal, it should be repeated serially over 7 to 14 days. If the test remains normal, it indicates that the patient either did not have a DVT or calf DVT which extended into the proximal veins, and therefore anticoagulant therapy can be withheld safely. Using the IPG, this approach has been validated in pregnant patients.[36]

VI. DIAGNOSTIC TESTS FOR DVT

Three tests which are useful for the diagnosis of DVT during pregnancy are IPG, CUS, and contrast venography. Studies published before 1990 suggest that the IPG is highly sensitive to detect proximal DVT in symptomatic out-patients. However, two recent studies from McMaster University suggest that the sensitivity of IPG for proximal DVT is much lower than reported earlier.[37,38] The lower sensitivity is probably due to the fact that patients with DVT are referred to the McMaster University-based hospitals with minimal symptoms, i.e. at a time when their thrombi are smaller, less likely to be occlusive and, therefore, less likely to cause an abnormal IPG. The safety of withholding anticoagulant therapy if serial IPG remains normal has been demonstrated in several clinical trials, including one in pregnant patients.[32-34,36] However, the results of a recent study in which a new IPG machine was used suggest that the thrombotic event rate (including deaths) is unacceptably high in patients with normal IPG.[39] It is not clear whether the high event rate reported in that study, was due to the insensitivity of the IPG machine used. Until further information becomes available, it seems reasonable to use IPG in conjunction with clinical likelihood; if the clinical likelihood is high but the IPG is normal, further testing should be performed (see below).

CUS is highly sensitive to proximal DVT in symptomatic out-patients.[35] The finding of a non-compressible venous segment has a very high positive predictive value for DVT. The safety of withholding anticoagulant therapy in non-pregnant patients, if serial CUS remains normal within 7 days of presentation, has been demonstrated in a large clinical trial.[35] Although CUS is highly sensitive and specific for thrombi in the common femoral, superficial femoral and popliteal veins, it may be insensitive to isolated iliac DVT. Indirect approaches such as measuring the diameter of the iliac vein or pulsed Doppler sampling of the common femoral vein may be more useful in detecting iliac vein thrombosis and should be considered if a patient presents with a clinical suspicion of iliac vein thrombosis (i.e. cramping, unilateral abdominal pain in conjunction with unilateral leg pain and swelling of the entire extremity).

Adequately performed contrast venography is the reference standard for the diagnosis of DVT.[31] A limited venogram can be performed in the pregnant patient, using pelvic and abdominal shielding with a lead-containing apron. This minimizes the amount of radiation absorbed by the fetus but does not allow visualization of the iliac vein.

A. AN APPROACH TO THE PATIENT WITH CLINICALLY SUSPECTED DVT DURING PREGNANCY

Either IPG or CUS can be used as the initial diagnostic test in pregnant patients with clinically suspected DVT (Figs. 1 and 2). If the IPG is abnormal during the first two trimesters, DVT can be diagnosed. If the IPG is abnormal during the third trimester, it may be falsely positive because of outflow obstruction caused by the gravid uterus and further investigation with a limited venogram or CUS should be considered. If either of these is also abnormal, DVT can be diagnosed. If a limited venogram is normal, a complete venogram should be performed to confirm whether or not the patient has iliac vein thrombosis. If the initial IPG is negative, serial IPG testing over 7 to 14 days should be performed. If the test becomes abnormal, DVT can be diagnosed, whereas if the test remains normal, a clinically important DVT can be excluded. Due to the recent concern about the sensitivity of IPG, consideration should be given to performing venography or CUS in a patient with a high pre-test likelihood of DVT and a normal initial IPG. If CUS is performed, the diagnostic algorithm in Fig. 2 can be followed.

CUS is a reasonable alternative to IPG as the initial diagnostic test. DVT can be diagnosed if the test is positive at any time during pregnancy. If the test is normal, calf DVT or isolated iliac DVT may still be the cause of the patient's symptoms. If the latter is clinically suspected, the indirect methods of evaluating the thrombotic status of the iliac vein by duplex should be considered. Alternatively, IPG, which should be sensitive to iliac DVT, or venography can be performed. If iliac DVT is not a consideration and the initial CUS is normal, serial CUS over 7 to 14 days should be performed.

If neither IPG nor CUS is available, venography should be performed, limited at first and, if normal, repeated with complete venography. It is our belief that the risks of clinical misdiagnosis are greater than the risks of performing contrast venography.

VII. DIAGNOSTIC TESTS FOR PE

The tests which are useful in the patient with a clinically suspected PE include ventilation perfusion lung scanning, pulmonary angiography,

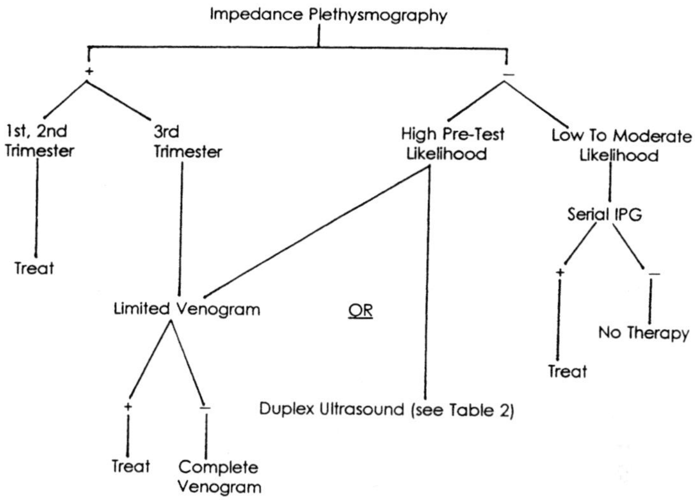

Figure 1. Algorithm using IPG for the management of pregnant patients with suspected DVT during pregnancy.

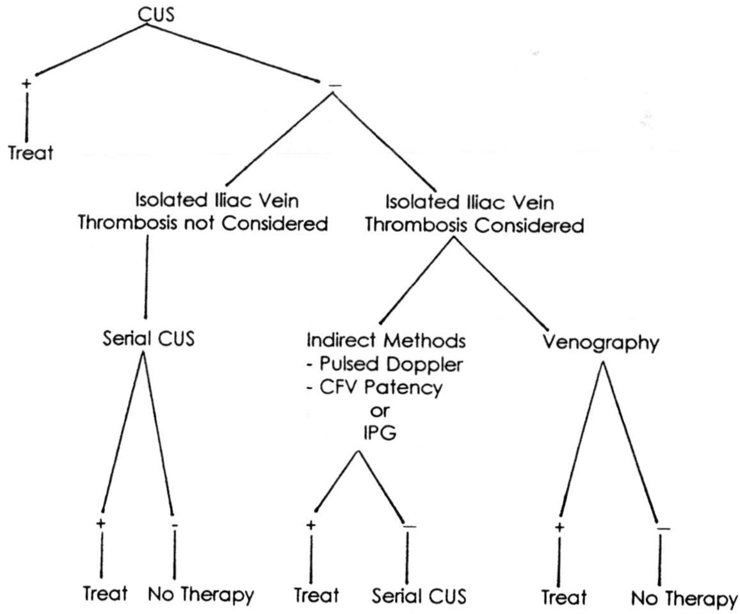

Figure 2. Algorithm using CUS for the management of pregnant patients with suspected DVT during pregnancy.

and the tests described above for the diagnosis of DVT. The latter are useful because DVT is present frequently in patients with PE, and because the detection of DVT in a patient with clinically suspected PE provides sufficient evidence to make a diagnosis of PE without performing additional tests.[40]

Although pulmonary angiography is the reference standard for the diagnosis of PE, it is invasive and expensive, and therefore is reserved for situations in which other less invasive tests are not diagnostic. Fetal radiation exposure should be minimized by using the brachial approach when possible and avoiding fluoroscopy over the pelvis when the femoral approach is used.

Ventilation perfusion lung scanning is currently the test of choice in patients with clinically suspected PE.[31] In non-pregnant patients, a normal perfusion scan excludes PE, whereas a high probability scan [segmental or large (>75% of the segment) subsegmental perfusion defect with normal ventilation] has a positive predictive value of approximately 90%. Approximately one half of non-pregnant patients with suspected PE have neither a normal perfusion scan nor a high probability lung scan; this type of scan result can be referred to as non-diagnostic or non-high. The prevalence of PE in patients with a non-high lung scan pattern is approximately 25%.[42] Therefore, in patients with non-high lung scans further investigation is indicated.

A. APPROACH TO THE PATIENT WITH CLINICALLY SUSPECTED PE DURING PREGNANCY

An approach to the pregnant patient with clinically suspected PE is summarized in Fig. 3. A chest radiograph is useful to exclude conditions such as fractured rib or pneumothorax that can cause symptoms similar to those seen with PE. Both a ventilation and a perfusion lung scan, using a reduced dose of radioisotope for the perfusion scan, are recommended. In some centres, a perfusion scan is performed alone as the initial test. The advantage of this approach is that if the perfusion scan is normal, PE can be excluded without the need for a ventilation scan. The disadvantage of this approach is that if the perfusion scan is abnormal, it is necessary to wait another 24 hours before the ventilation scan can be performed. In some centres, it may be easier to perform a non-invasive test of the legs, such as IPG or CUS. These tests are useful only if positive, since it is reasonable to diagnose PE in a patient with suspected PE who has an abnormal IPG or CUS. However, a normal IPG or CUS does not exclude PE, and, if this occurs, further investigation with a lung scan is indicated.

If the results of the perfusion scan are normal, PE can be

excluded.[43] If the lung scan is a high probability, particularly in patients with a high or moderate pre-test likelihood, PE can be diagnosed.[41] In non-pregnant patients with a low pre-test likelihood and a high probability lung scan, the post-test likelihood for PE is approximately 50-60%.[44] In pregnant patients, this combination may be associated with a higher post-test likelihood of PE than in pregnant patients because pregnant patients are less likely to have co-morbid conditions that could cause an abnormal lung scan. Nevertheless, it may be reasonable to perform pulmonary angiography in selected pregnant patients with a low pre-test likelihood of PE and a high probability lung scan, such as those with a contraindication to heparin.

In patients with a non-diagnostic lung scan, further investigation is indicated. IPG or CUS can be performed and the patient treated if the results are abnormal. However, if the results are normal, a pulmonary angiogram should be strongly considered. An approach that has been validated in non-pregnant patients with non-high scans is the performance of serial IPG over 14 days and withholding anticoagulants if the results are normal.[45] This approach has not been evaluated in pregnant patients and, therefore, cannot be recommended.

VIII. TREATMENT OF DVT/PE DURING PREGNANCY

The use of anticoagulants during pregnancy is problematic because of the potential side-effects to the mother and the fetus. Heparin does not cross the placenta[46] and is not expected to produce adverse fetal effects whereas warfarin crosses the placenta and is potentially teratogenic.[47] The safety of heparin and oral anticoagulant therapy has recently been reviewed; it is likely that heparin is safe for the fetus, whereas oral anticoagulants may not be.[48,49]

A. HEPARIN

Contrary to a previous report[50], it was suggested in a recent critical review of the literature of heparin therapy during pregnancy[48], that heparin therapy is safe for the fetus. This conclusion has been supported in a cohort study of 100 pregnancies in which the rates of prematurity, spontaneous abortions, stillbirths, neonatal deaths and congenital malformations associated with heparin therapy were comparable to the normal population.[49]

Side-effects of heparin include bleeding, thrombocytopenia and osteoporosis. The reported frequency of bleeding with heparin

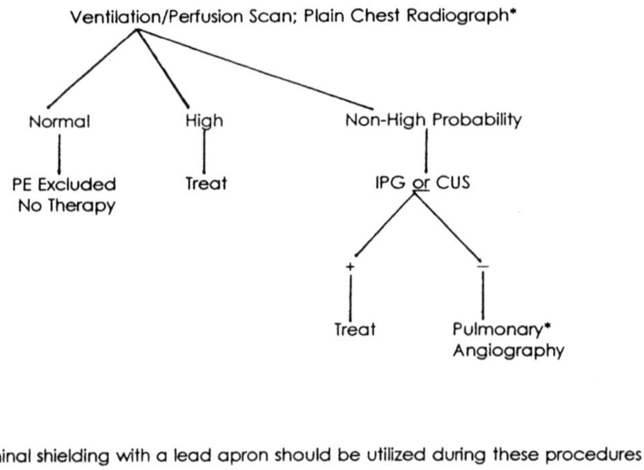

Figure 3. Algorithm for the management of pregnant patients with suspected PE.

therapy during pregnancy was 2% in the above mentioned cohort study.[49] This is similar to the rate observed in non-pregnant patients receiving heparin.[50,64] There is no increased bleeding risk for the fetus since heparin does not cross the placenta.

In a recent cohort study of 11 pregnancies in 10 pregnant women receiving adjusted dose subcutaneous heparin therapy at the time of delivery, it was reported that an anticoagulant effect persisted for up to 28 hours after the last injection of heparin.[51] As a result, in women who were being treated with adjusted dose subcutaneous heparin, the delivery was frequently complicated by a prolonged aPTT which is associated with an increased risk of bleeding. The mechanism for this prolonged anticoagulant effect is unclear. However, one way of avoiding an unwanted anticoagulant effect during delivery is to discontinue heparin therapy 24 hours prior to elective induction of labour. This should avoid the problem of having an anticoagulant effect at the time of delivery, thereby reducing the risk of bleeding. If an anticoagulant effect occurs at the time of delivery, judicious use of protamine sulfate to neutralize the heparin should be considered.

Heparin-induced thrombocytopenia is usually associated with a fall in the platelet count 6 to 12 days after the initiation of heparin.[52] This syndrome occurs more commonly with bovine-derived than with porcine-derived heparin[53] and paradoxically, can be associated with thrombotic problems. When this complication occurs, heparin should be discontinued.

Long-term heparin therapy has been reported to cause osteoporosis in both laboratory animals and humans, but the underlying mechanism for this is unknown. Two recent studies have provided estimates of the risk of symptomatic fractures in patients treated with long-term heparin therapy.[54,55] In the first study[54], a cohort of 61 consecutive pre-menopausal women previously treated with long-term heparin were compared with a group of controls matched for age, parity, and duration between the last pregnancy. The patients were interviewed to determine the incidence of symptomatic fractures and were evaluated with dual photon absorptiometry of the lumbar spine and single photon absorptiometry of the wrist in order to detect any sub-clinical reduction of bone density. None of the heparin-treated patients had suffered a symptomatic fracture (0 of 61, 95% confidence intervals 0.0 to 5.9%), but there was a significantly greater proportion of heparin-treated patients than controls who had reduced bone density. In the second study[55], 70 patients treated with subcutaneous heparin therapy during pregnancy underwent X-ray of the spine and hip immediately post-partum and again at 6 to 12 months post-partum. There were 12 patients with osteopenia and 2 patients with multiple fractures of the spine. Re-examination at 6 to 12 months post partum demonstrated that the changes were reversible in most cases. It can be concluded from these 2 studies that a subclinical reduction in bone density can occur as a consequence of long-term heparin therapy, although the risk of symptomatic fractures is low. It is unknown whether women who suffer a subclinical reduction in bone density due to heparin are predisposed to fractures in the post-menopausal period.

It is likely that the risk of osteoporosis is dependent upon the dose of heparin used and the duration of heparin therapy. It is not known whether supplemental calcium prevents the reduction of bone density that occurs in women receiving long-term heparin therapy but it seems reasonable to use it empirically.

Heparin must be administered parenterally and during pregnancy, heparin is usually administered by subcutaneous (SC) injection twice daily. The use of an indwelling subcutaneous Teflon catheter that must be replaced on a weekly basis may improve the tolerability of long-term heparin administration during pregnancy.[56]

B. WARFARIN

Warfarin exposure between 6 and 12 weeks of gestation can be associated with warfarin embryopathy which is characterized by stippled epiphyses and nasal hypoplasia.[47] Central nervous abnormalities, both hemorrhage and malformations, have been reported after warfarin exposure at any time during pregnancy but the incidence appears to be low.[48] Therefore, heparin currently is the anticoagulant of choice during pregnancy. If warfarin is used, it should be restricted to the second and early third trimesters and should be avoided between 6 and 12 weeks of gestation and near term in order to avoid the delivery of an anticoagulated fetus.

C. TREATMENT OF ACUTE DVT/PE DURING PREGNANCY

Heparin is usually initiated with an intravenous (IV) bolus of 5000 units followed by a maintenance dose administered as a continuous IV infusion of 24,000-32,000 units/24 hours in order to prolong aPTT into the therapeutic range (usually 2 to 3 times the control). Adjusted dose heparin is comparable to IV heparin in both efficacy and safety, provided a sufficient dose is used (usually 30-40,000 units/day in 2 divided doses).[57,58] At the present time, SC heparin should be reserved for situations in which IV heparin cannot be administered. Recent studies have demonstrated that 4 to 5 days of IV heparin is adequate initial therapy for DVT.[59-61] After the initial IV heparin, SC heparin should be administered 12 hourly in doses adjusted to prolong a 6 hour post-injection aPTT to approximately 2 to 3 times control. The aPTT should be checked regularly since the heparin requirements may vary as pregnancy progresses. Anticoagulant therapy should probably be continued throughout pregnancy and for 4 to 6 weeks after the delivery.

D. PATIENTS RECEIVING LONG-TERM ANTICOAGULANT THERAPY PRIOR TO PREGNANCY

Patients who are receiving warfarin prior to pregnancy for DVT/PE or for the prevention of systemic embolism should be treated with 12 hourly SC heparin throughout pregnancy in doses adjusted to prolong the 6 hours post-injection aPTT to approximately 2 to 3 times control. Two options are available when patients receiving long-term anticoagulant therapy decide to conceive. The first option is to switch to heparin before conception. This has the advantage of avoiding any exposure of the fetus to warfarin therapy but increases the duration of heparin exposure if conception is delayed. The second option is to continue warfarin and perform regular pregnancy tests when conception is attempted. As soon as the pregnancy test becomes positive, warfarin should be stopped and heparin commenced. This is probably safe for the fetus, provided warfarin is discontinued prior to 6 weeks of gestation. As mentioned previously, no cases of fetal embryopathy have been described with warfarin exposure prior to 6 weeks of gestation.[62] Warfarin therapy can be resumed after the delivery.

E. PREVIOUS DVT/PE

The optimal management of pregnant patients with previous DVT/PE is unknown because there are no large prospective trials to provide reliable estimates of the incidence and timing of recurrence during pregnancy. It is our belief that until such estimates are available, some form of prophylaxis or surveillance should be instituted. It had been our practice to administer heparin 5000 units every 12 hours throughout the pregnancy in women with previous DVT or PE.[63] Surveillance with weekly IPG or duplex ultrasonography may be a reasonable alternative to heparin during pregnancy.[63]

F. DELIVERY AND POST-PARTUM

If the patient is receiving heparin 5000 units every 12 hours at term, heparin can be discontinued at the onset of true labor. No increase in bleeding is anticipated with this approach. As discussed above, if adjusted dose heparin is being administered at term, there is a strong possibility that the delivery will occur in the presence of a prolonged aPTT, which may, in turn, be associated with an increase in bleeding complications. To overcome this problem, it is now our practice to electively induce labor in women who are receiving adjusted dose heparin; heparin therapy is discontinued 24 hours prior to induction. Most patients will have a normal aPTT at the time of the delivery with this approach. In patients who are considered to be at high risk for thrombotic complications, an IV heparin infusion can be started after discontinuation of SC heparin. Since the half-life of IV heparin is short[64], heparin can be discontinued 4 to 6 hours before delivery with the expectation that the aPTT will be normal at the time of delivery.

After delivery, heparin should be restarted as soon as hemostasis is obtained (usually 2-12 hours) and warfarin therapy can be started the same day. Heparin can be discontinued when warfarin has reached a therapeutic level [international normalized ratio (INR) of 2-3] for 2 consecutive days. This is because the initial prolongation of the INR is due largely to a decrement in the levels of Factor VII which has the shortest half-life of the vitamin K-dependent clotting factors, but is unlikely to indicate an optimal antithrombotic effect. Warfarin and heparin are both safe for the breast-fed infant when administered to the nursing mother.[65,66]

IX. INHERITED MOLECULAR DEFICIENCIES

Deficiencies of antithrombin III, protein C and protein S have autosomal dominant inheritance and the presence of any of these is associated with an increased risk of thrombosis.[67-69] The correct approach to pregnant patients with one of these deficiencies is unknown because the true risk of venous thrombosis in pregnant women with antithrombin III, Protein C or Protein S deficiency has not been studied in appropriately designed trials. Patients with these deficiencies and previous VTE will often be receiving long-term anticoagulant therapy. In such patients, warfarin should be replaced by adjusted-dose heparin prior to 6 weeks of gestation. The optimal management of asymptomatic patients with these deficiencies, most of whom are not receiving long-term anticoagulant therapy, is unknown. A recent study suggests that the incidence of antepartum thrombosis (diagnosed on clinical grounds in 78 pregnant women with either antithrombin III, protein C or protein S deficiency[70]) is 14%, 4% and 0%, respectively, and post-partum thrombosis (diagnosed on clinical grounds) is 28%, 18% and 17%, respectively. This study suggests that anticoagulant prophylaxis is justified during the post-partum period in antithrombin III, Protein C and Protein S deficient individuals. However, it is not clear whether anticoagulant prophylaxis is required during pregnancy, especially for protein S deficient patients. It has been our practice either to administer low-dose heparin throughout pregnancy or to perform frequent surveillance with IPG or duplex ultrasonography in asymptomatic Protein C and Protein S deficient individuals. In antithrombin III deficient patients, pregnancy has been managed successfully using either heparin alone[71,72] or a combination of heparin and antithrombin III concentrate.[73-76] It has been a concern that the risk of VTE may be higher in antithrombin III deficient patients treated with heparin since heparin may cause antithrombin III levels to decrease even further. Therefore, antithrombin III concentrate may theoretically be a useful adjunct to heparin therapy. However, the role of antithrombin III concentrate during pregnancy and at delivery is still unknown.[74] Antithrombin III concentrate is a blood product and carries the potential risk of viral transmission. Therefore, it should probably be reserved for antithrombin III deficient patients who have heparin resistance or thromboembolic recurrence despite adequate heparin therapy.

REFERENCES

1. **Kaunitz, A.M., Hughes, J.M., Grimes, D.A., Smith, J.C., Rochat, R.W., Kafrissen, M.E.** Causes of maternal mortality in the United States. *Obstet Gynecol* 65, 605, 1985.
2. **Sacks, B.P., Brown, D.A. J., Driscoll, S.G., Schulman, E., Acker, D., Ransil, B.J., Jewett, J.F.** Maternal mortality in

Massachusetts. Trends and prevention. *N Engl J Med* 316, 667, 1987.

3. **Goodrich, S.M., Wood, J.E.** Peripheral venous distensibility and velocity of venous blood flow during pregnancy or during oral contraceptive therapy. *Am J Obstet Gynecol* 90, 740, 1964.
4. **Ikard, R.W., Ueland, K., Folse, R.** Lower limb venous dynamics in pregnant women. *Surg Gynecol Obstet* 132, 483, 1971.
5. **Kerr, M.G., Scott, D.B., Samuel, E.** Studies of the inferior vena cava in late pregnancy. *Br Med J* 1, 532, 1964.
6. **Stirling, Y., Woolf, L., North, W.R.S., Seghatchian, M.J., Meade, T.W.** Haemostasis in normal pregnancy. *Thromb Haemost* 52, 176, 1984.
7. **Reid, D.E., Frigoletto, F.D., Tullis, J.L., Hinman, J.** Hypercoagulable states in pregnancy. *Am J Obstet Gynecol* 111, 493, 1971.
8. **Weenink, G.H., Treffers, P.E., Kahlé, L.H., ten Cate, J.W.** Antithrombin III in normal pregnancy. *Thromb Res* 26, 281, 1982.
9. **Weiner, C.P., Brandt, J.** Plasma antithrombin III activity in normal pregnancy. *Obstet Gynecol* 56, 601, 1980.
10. **de Boer, K., ten Cate, J.W., Sturk, A., Borm J.J.J., Treffers P.E.** Enhanced thrombin generation in normal and hypertensive pregnancy. *Am J Obstet Gynecol* 160, 95, 1989.
11. **Gjonnaess, H., Fagerhol, M.K.** Studies on coagulation and fibrinolysis in pregnancy. *Acta Obstet Gynecol Scand* 54, 363, 1975.
12. **Gonzalez, R., Alberca, I., Vicente, V.** Protein C levels in late pregnancy, post-partum and in women on oral contraceptives. *Thromb Res* 39, 637, 1985.
13. **Comp, P.C., Thurnau, G.R., Welsh, J., Esmon, C.T.** Functional and immunologic protein S levels are decreased during pregnancy. *Blood* 68, 881, 1986.
14. **Weiner, C.P., Kwaan, H., Hauck, W.W., Duboe, F.J., Paul, M., Wallemark, C-B.** Fibrin generation in normal pregnancy. *Obstet Gynecol* 64, 46, 1984.
15. **Bonnar, J., McNicol, G.P., Douglas, A.S.** Coagulation and fibrinolytic mechanisms during and after normal childbirth. *Br Med J* 2, 200, 1970.
16. **Ygge, J.** Changes in blood coagulation and fibrinolysis during the puerperium. *Am J Obstet Gynecol* 104, 2, 1969.
17. **Wright, J.G., Cooper, P., Astedt, B., Lecander, I., Wilde, J.T., Preston, F.E., Greaves, M.** Fibrinolysis during normal human pregnancy: complex inter-relationships between plasma levels

of tissue plasminogen activator and inhibitors and the euglobulin clot lysis time. *Br J Haematol* 69, 253, 1988.
18. **Kruithof, E.K.O., Tran-Thang, C., Gudinchet, A., Hauert, J., Nicoloso, G., Genton, C., Welti, H., Bachmann, F.** Fibrinolysis in pregnancy: A study of plasminogen activator inhibitors. *Blood* 69, 460, 1987.
19. **Ballegeer, V., Mombaerts, P., Declerck, P.J., Spitz, B., Van Assche, F.A., Collen, D.** Fibrinolytic response to venous occlusion and fibrin fragment D-Dimer levels in normal and complicated pregnancy. *Thromb Haemost* 58, 1030, 1987.
20. **Mackinnon, S., Walker, I.D., Davidson, J.F., Walker, J.J.** Plasma fibrinolysis during and after normal childbirth. *Br J Haemat* 65, 339, 1987.
21. **Gordon, Y.B., Ratky, S.M., Sola, C.M., Lewis, J., Baker, L.R.I., Chard, T.** Circulating levels of fibrin/fibrinogen degradation fragment E in normal pregnancy and in association with intrauterine growth retardation and perinatal asphyxia. *Br J Obs Gyn* 82, 958, 1975.
22. **Andrew, M., Mitchell, L., Berry, L., Paes, B., Delorme, M., Ofosu, F., Burrows, R., Khamballa, B.** An anticoagulant dermatan sulfate proteoglycan circulates in the pregnant woman and her fetus. *J Clin Invest* 89, 321, 1992.
23. **Drill, V.A., Calhoun, D.W.** Oral contraceptives and thromboembolic disease. *JAMA* 206, 77, 1968.
24. **Kierkegaard, A.** Incidence and diagnosis of deep vein thrombosis associated with pregnancy. *Acta Obstet Gynecol Scand* 62, 39, 1983.
25. **Bergqvist, A., Bergqvist, D., Hallbook, T.** Deep vein thrombosis during pregnancy: A prospective study. *Acta Obstet Gynecol Scand* 62, 443, 1983
26. **Ginsberg, J.S., Brill-Edwards, P., Bona, R., Burrows, R.** Deep vein thrombosis (DVT) during pregnancy: leg and trimester of presentation. *Thromb Haemost* 67, 519, 1992.
27. **Cockett, F.B., Thomas, M.L.** The iliac compression syndrome. *Br J Surg* 52, 816, 1965.
28. **Huisman, M.V., Buller, H.R., ten Cate, J.W., van Royen, E.A., Vreeken, J., Kersten, M-J., Bakx, R.** Unexpected high prevalence of silent pulmonary embolism in patients with deep venous thrombosis. *Chest* 95, 498, 1989.
29. **Ginsberg, J.S., Hirsh, J., Rainbow, A.J., Coates, J.** Risks to the fetus of radiologic procedures used in the diagnosis of maternal venous thromboembolic disease. *Thromb Haemost* 61, 189, 1989.
30. **Wells, P.S., Anderson, D.R., Kearon, C., Weitz, J.I., Hirsh, J.**

The combination of pre-test clinical likelihood and non-invasive tests improves the management of out-patients with suspected deep vein thrombosis. *Thromb Haemost* 69s, 1080, 1993.

31. **Hull, R.D. Raskob, G.E., Leclerc, J.R., Jay, R.M., Hirsh, J.** The diagnosis of clinically suspected venous thrombosis. *Clin Chest Med* 5, 439, 1984.
32. **Huisman, M.V., Buller, H.R., ten Cate, J.W., Heijermans, H.S.F., van der Laan, J., van Maanen, D.J.** Management of clinically suspected acute venous thrombosis in outpatients with serial impedance plethysmography in a community hospital setting. *Arch Intern Med* 149, 511, 1989.
33. **Huisman, M.V., Buller, H.R., ten Cate, J.W., Vreeken, J.** Serial impedance plethysmography for suspected deep venous thrombosis in outpatients. *N Engl J Med* 314, 823, 1986.
34. **Hull, R.D., Hirsh, J., Carter, C.J.** Diagnostic efficacy of impedance plethysmography for clinically suspected deep-vein thrombosis: a randomized trial. *Ann Intern Med* 102, 21, 1985.
35. **Heijboer, H., Brandjes, D.P.M., Lensing, A.W.A., Buller, H.R., ten Cate, J.W.** Efficacy of real-time B-mode ultrasonography versus impedance plethysmography in the diagnosis of deep-vein thrombosis in symptomatic outpatients. *N Engl J Med* 329, 1365, 1993.
36. **Hull, R.D., Raskob, G.E., Carter, C.J.** Serial impedance plethysmography in pregnant patients with clinically suspected deep-vein thrombosis. Clinical validity of negative findings. *Ann Intern Med* 112, 663, 1990.
37. **Anderson, D.R., Lensing, A.W.A., Wells, P.S., Levine, M.N., Weitz, J.I., Hirsh, J.** Limitations of impedance plethysmography in the diagnosis of clinically suspected deep-vein thrombosis. *Ann Intern Med* 118, 25, 1993.
38. **Ginsberg, J.S., Wells, P.S., Hirsh, J., Panju, A.A., Patel, M.A., Malone, D.E., McGinnis, J., Stevens, P., Brill-Edwards, P.** Reevaluation of the sensitivity of impedance plethysmography for the detection of proximal deep vein thrombosis. *Arch Intern Med* In press, 1994.
39. **Prandoni, P., Lensing, A.W.A., Buller, H.R., Carta, M., Vigo, M., Cogo, A., Cuppini, S., ten Cate, J.W.** Failure of computerized impedance plethysmography in the diagnostic management of patients with clinically suspected deep vein thrombosis. *Thromb Haemost* 65, 233, 1991.
40. **Hull, R.D., Hirsh, J., Carter, C.J., Jay, R.M., Dodd, P.E., Ockelford, P.A., Coates, G., Gill, G.J., Turpie, A.G.G., Doyle, D.J., Buller, H.R., Raskob G.E.** Pulmonary angiography, ventilation lung scanning and venography for clinically

suspected pulmonary embolism with abnormal perfusion lung scan. *Ann Intern Med* 98, 891, 1983.

41. **Hull, R.D., Hirsh, J., Carter, C.J., Raskob, G.E., Gill, G.J., Jay, R.M., Leclerc, J.R., David, M., Coates, G.** Diagnostic value of ventilation-perfusion lung scanning in patients with suspected pulmonary embolism. *Chest* 88, 819, 1985
42. **Hull, R.D., Raskob, G.E., Hirsh, J.** The diagnosis of clinically suspected pulmonary embolism. *Chest* 89, 417s, 1986
43. **Hull, R.D., Raskob, G.E., Coates, G., Panju, A.A.** Clinical validity of a normal perfusion lung scan in patients with suspected pulmonary embolism. *Chest* 97, 23, 1990.
44. **The PIOPED Investigators.** Value of the ventilation/perfusion scan in acute pulmonary embolism. Results of the prospective investigation of pulmonary embolism diagnosis (PIOPED). *JAMA* 263, 2753, 1990.
45. **Hull, R.D., Raskob, G., Coates, G., Panju, A.A., Gill, G.J.** A new noninvasive management strategy for patients with suspected pulmonary embolism. *Arch Intern Med* 149, 2549, 1989.
46. **Flessa, H.C., Kapstrom, A.B., Glueck, H.I., Will, J.J.** Placental transport of heparin. *Am J Obstet Gynecol* 93, 570, 1965.
47. **Becker, M.H., Genieser, N.B., Finegold, M., Miranda, D., Spackman, T.** Chondrodysplasia punctata. Is maternal warfarin therapy a factor? *Am J Dis Child* 129, 356, 1975
48. **Ginsberg, J.S., Hirsh, J., Turner, D.C., Levine, M.N., Burrows, R.** Risks to the fetus of anticoagulant therapy during pregnancy. *Thromb Haemost* 61, 197, 1989.
49. **Ginsberg, J.S., Kowalchuk, G., Hirsh, J., Brill-Edwards, P., Burrows, R.** Heparin therapy during pregnancy: Risks to the fetus and mother. *Arch Intern Med* 149, 2233, 1989.
50. **Hull, R., Delore, T., Carter, C., Hirsh, J., Genton, E., Gent, M., Turpie, G., McLaughlin, D.** Adjusted subcutaneous heparin versus warfarin sodium in the long-term treatment of venous thrombosis. *N Engl J Med* 306, 189, 1982.
51. **Anderson, D.R., Ginsberg, J.S., Burrows, R., Brill-Edwards, P.** Subcutaneous heparin therapy during pregnancy: a need for concern at the time of delivery. *Thromb Haemost* 65, 248, 1991
52. **King, D.J., Kelton, J.G.** Heparin-associated thrombocytopenia. *Ann Intern Med* 100, 535, 1984
53. **Powers, P.J., Kelton, J.G., Carter, C.J.** Studies on the frequency of heparin-associated thrombocytopenia. *Thromb Res* 33, 439, 1984.
54. **Ginsberg, J.S., Kowalchuk, G., Hirsh, J., Brill-Edwards, P.,**

Burrows, R., Coates, G., Webber, C. Heparin effect on bone density. *Thromb Haemost* 64, 286, 1990

55. **Dahlman, T., Sjoberg, H.E., Hellgren, M., Bucht, E.** Calcium homeostasis in pregnancy during long-term heparin treatment. *Br J Obstet Gynaecol* 99, 412, 1992.
56. **Anderson, D.R., Ginsberg, J., Brill-Edwards, P., Demers, C., Grant, B., Hirsh, J.** Teflon catheter use for subcutaneous heparin administration during pregnancy: A randomized crossover study. *Arch Intern Med* 153, 841, 1993.
57. **Andersson, G., Fagrell, B., Holmgren, K., Johnsson, H., Ljungberg, B., Nilsson, E., Wilhelmsson, S., Zetterquist, S.** Subcutaneous administration of heparin; a randomised comparison with intravenous administration of heparin to patients with deep-vein thrombosis. *Thromb Res* 27, 631, 1982
58. **Hommes, D.W., Bura, A., Mazzolai, L., Buller, H.R., ten Cate, J.W.** Subcutaneous heparin compared to continuous intravenous heparin administration in the initial treatment of deep vein thrombosis: A systematic overview and meta-analysis. *Thromb Haemost* 65, 753a, 1991.
59. **Hull, R.D., Raskob, G.E., Rosenbloom, D., Panju, A.A., Brill-Edwards, P., Ginsberg, J.S., Hirsh, J., Martin, G.J., Green, D.** Heparin for 5 days as compared with 10 days in the initial treatment of proximal venous thrombosis. *N Engl J Med* 322, 1260, 1990.
60. **Schulman, S., Lockner, D., Bergstrom, K., Blomback, M.** Intensive initial oral anticoagulation and shorter heparin treatment in deep venous thrombosis. *Thromb Haemost* 52, 276, 1984
61. **Gallus, A., Jackaman, J., Tillett, J., Mills, W., Wycherley, A.** Safety and efficacy of warfarin started early after submassive venous thrombosis or pulmonary embolism. *Lancet* 2, 1293, 1986
62. **Iturbe-Alessio, I., Del Carmen Fonseca, M., Mutchinik, O., Santos, M.A., Zajarias, A., Salazar, E.** Risks of anticoagulant therapy in pregnant women with artifical heart valves. *N Engl J Med* 315, 1390, 1986
63. **Ginsberg, J.S., Hirsh, J.** Use of antithrombotic agents during pregnancy. *Chest* 102, 385, 1992
64. **Hirsh, J., Van Aken, W.G., Gallus, A.S., Dollery, C.T., Cade, J.F., Yung, W.L.** Heparin kinetics in venous thrombosis and pulmonary embolism. *Circ* 53, 691, 1976.
65. **Orme, M.L'e, Lewis, P.J., De Swiet, M., Serlin, M.J., Sibeon, R., Baty, J.D., Breckenridge, A.M.** May mothers given warfarin breast-feed their infants? *Br Med J* 1, 1564, 1977.

66. **McKenna, R., Cole, E.R., Vasan, U.** Is warfarin sodium contraindicated in the lactating mother? *J Pediatr* 103, 325, 1983.
67. **Thaler, E., Lechner, K.** Antithrombin III deficiency in thromboembolism. *Clin Haematol* 10, 369, 1981.
68. **Broekmans, A.W., Veltkamp, J.J., Bertina, R.M.** Congenital protein C deficiency and venous thromboembolism: a study of three Dutch families. *N Engl J Med* 309, 340, 1983.
69. **Kamiya, T., Sugihara, T., Ogata, K., Saito, H., Suzuki, K., Nishioka, J., Hashimoto, S., Yamagata, K.** Inherited deficiency of protein S in a Japanese family with recurrent venous thrombosis: A study of three generations. *Blood* 67, 406, 1986.
70. **Conard, J., Horellou, M.H., Van Dreden, P., Lecompte, T., Samama, M.** Thrombosis and pregnancy in congenital deficiencies in ATIII, Protein C or Protein S: A study of 78 women. *Thromb Haemost* 63, 319, 1990
71. **Leclerc, J.R., Geerts, W., Panju, A., Nguyen, P., Hirsh, J.** Management of anti-thrombin III deficiency during pregnancy without administration of anti-thrombin III. *Thromb Res* 41, 567, 1986.
72. **Brandt, P., Stenbjerg, S.** Subcutaneous heparin for thrombosis in pregnant women with hereditary antithrombin deficiency. *Lancet* 1, 100, 1979.
73. **Samson, D., Stirling, Y., Woolf, L., Howarth, D., Seghatchian, M.J., De Chazal, R.** Management of planned pregnancy in a patient with congenital antitrombin III deficiency. *Br J Haematol* 56, 243, 1984.
74. **Schwartz, R.S., Bauer, K.A., Rosenberg, R.D, Kavanaugh, E.J., Davies, D.C., Bogdanoff, D.A.** Clinical experience with antithrombin III concentrate in treatment of congenital and acquired deficiency of antithrombin. *Am J Med* 87(3B), 53S, 1989.
75. **Brandt, P.** Observations during the treatment of antithrombin-III deficient women with heparin and antithrombin concentrate during pregnancy, parturition and abortion. *Thromb Res* 22, 15, 1981.
76. **Hellgren, M., Tengborn, L., Abildgaard, U.** Pregnancy in women with congenital antithrombin III deficiency: Experience of treatment with heparin and antithrombin. *Gynecol Obstet Invest* 14, 127, 1982.

Chapter 10

THE HYPERCOAGULABLE STATE IN CANCER: INCREASED THROMBIN GENERATION AND IMPAIRED THROMBIN INHIBITION

A. Falanga, S. Cortelazzo and T. Barbui

I. INTRODUCTION

Thrombohemorrhagic disorders are frequent complications of malignant disease.[1,2] In addition, even in the absence of clinical symptoms, abnormalities of laboratory tests of hemostasis showing an activation of the clotting system are common features in patients with cancer.[3] These observations have been confirmed in experimental animal models[4,6] and provide evidence that malignancy is associated with a hypercoagulable state of the host.

The process of tumor growth and dissemination also is influenced by the mechanisms of fibrin formation and deposition.[1,2] Fibrin deposits have been demonstrated in and around the primary tumor burden and fibrin threads have been shown on the surface of disseminated potentially metastatic tumor cells.[7,10] The presence of a fibrin coat is considered to favour the metastatic process by inducing tumor cells and platelet clumps with subsequent obstruction of the microcirculation and extravasation.[11,12] This is also supported by the reports of anticoagulant and fibrinolytic agents being effective in reducing tumor growth and metastases in some experimental models.[5,13] This overview will focus on the mechanisms underlying these processes and their modulation by anticoagulant therapy.

II. PREVALENCE OF HEMOSTATIC DISORDERS IN CANCER

The association of malignant disease with an increased risk of thromboembolic disorders (TED) has been well recognized for more than 120 years.[1] Since then, a variety of thrombohemorrhagic complications have been described in malignancy, including both venous and arterial thrombosis, migratory thrombophlebitis, pulmonary embolism, non-bacterial thrombotic endocarditis, and disseminated intravascular coagulation (DIC). The overall prevalence of these complications varied between 1% and 11% according to earlier reports, although post-mortem studies suggest that these numbers are higher.[2]

Many variables can influence the association between TED and cancer, e.g. the type of tumor, the anti-cancer treatment, and the

0-8493-7649-1/95/$0.00+$.50

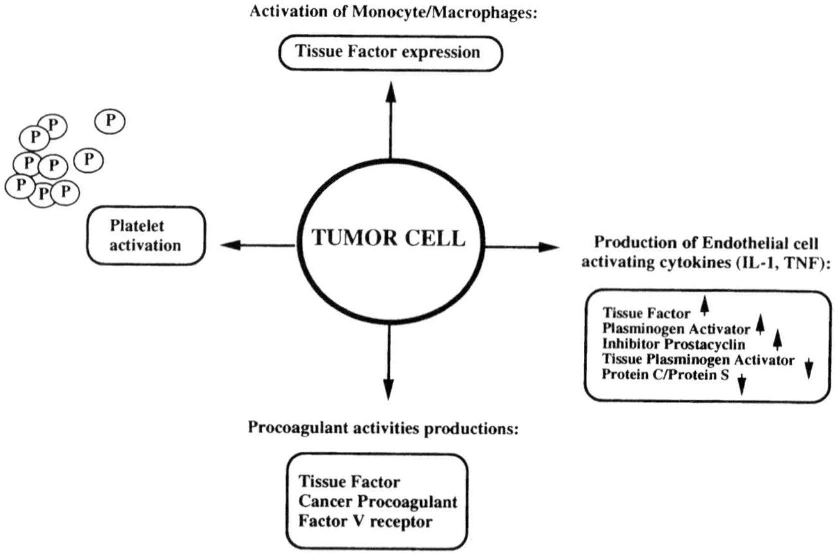

Figure 1. Schematics of the prinicpal mechanisms of tumor cell interaction with the hemostatic system.

objective criteria used for the diagnosis of thrombosis.

Mucin-secreting tumors of the gastrointestinal tract historically have been associated with the highest risk of TED[2,14,15]; however, a high incidence is reported for other types of tumors, e.g. pancreatic tumors (50%) and chronic myeloproliferative disorders (10-30%).[16,18] In addition, there is a peculiar distribution of the hemostatic disturbances. Thromboembolism is most frequent in solid tumors, while severe coagulopathy with bleeding diathesis, e.g., DIC, is most commonly associated with acute leukemias[19-21], particularly acute promyelocytic leukemia (APL) accounting for about 10% of early deaths in APL patients.[22] Further, it is now well established that anti-cancer therapy, including both surgery and chemotherapy, can contribute to the risk of thrombohemorrhagic complications. Post-operative deep vein thrombosis (DVT) is more frequent in patients with malignancy than in those operated on for non-malignant diseases.[23,24] Chemotherapeutic agents and hormones significantly increase the occurrence of thromboembolism in solid tumors[25] and exacerbate the bleeding of acute leukemia.[21] Clinical pictures of thrombosis have been described in association with specific anti-tumor drugs, i.e. L-asparaginase, mytomycin C, cysplatin and high dose conditioning treatments for bone marrow transplants.[26] Direct evidence of the thrombogenic effect of anti-cancer therapy has been provided by a prospective study of women with stage II breast cancer in which the incidence of thrombosis was 6.8% during treatment and no episodes occurring during the observation period without treatment.[25]

Using objective criteria and improved techniques for the diagnosis of venous thrombosis, studies have also been conducted to demonstrate whether a thrombotic event can precede the diagnosis of cancer, acting as a clinical manifestation of an otherwise occult malignancy. A recent prospective study has shown a significant incidence of a subsequent symptomatic cancer in patients with idiopathic venous thromboembolism. The calculated risk for a patient with idiopathic thrombosis having cancer was 7.6% and increased up to 17.1% in patients with recurrent thrombosis.[27]

III. ABNORMALITIES OF CLOTTING TESTS IN CANCER

A. EVIDENCE FOR INCREASED THROMBIN GENERATION

The body of evidence emerging by clinical observations has suggested an abnormal activation of blood coagulation in cancer patients. Possible contributory causes for TED in cancer include the capacity of tumor cells and their products to activate the coagulation and fibrinolytic systems, as well as interacting with platelets, leukocytes and endothelial cells (Fig. 1). In particular, tumor procoagulants, including tissue factor and cancer procoagulant, play an important role in the clot-promoting mechanisms.[28-30]

Several studies have documented significant alterations of one or more of the so-called "routine" clotting tests in up to 90% of patients with solid tumors and leukemias.[3,31] The most common abnormalities are an elevation in clotting factors (i.e. fibrinogen and Factors V, VIII, IX and XI), an elevated level of fibrinogen/fibrin degradation products (FDPs), and thrombocytosis. New tests for detecting the by-products of clotting reactions and proteinase-inhibitor complexes generated have become available and have helped provide a biochemical definition of the "prethrombotic state".[32] Specifically, the intrinsic and the tissue Factor/Factor VII pathways activate Factor X to generate Factor Xa and an inactive peptide, the Factor X activation peptide (Fig. 2, see next page). Incorporated subsequently into prothrombinase, the enzyme Factor Xa converts prothrombin to equimolar concentrations of thrombin and prothrombin fragment 1+2 (F1+2). Thus, the thrombin produced either interacts with its major plasma substrate, fibrinogen (to form soluble fibrin monomers and fibrinopeptides A and B [FPA & B], and ultimately cross-links fibrin), or thrombin becomes inactivated by its major plasma inhibitors antithrombin III (ATIII) and heparin cofactor II (HCII) [as evidenced by the formation of circulating thrombin-ATIII (TAT) and thrombin-HCII

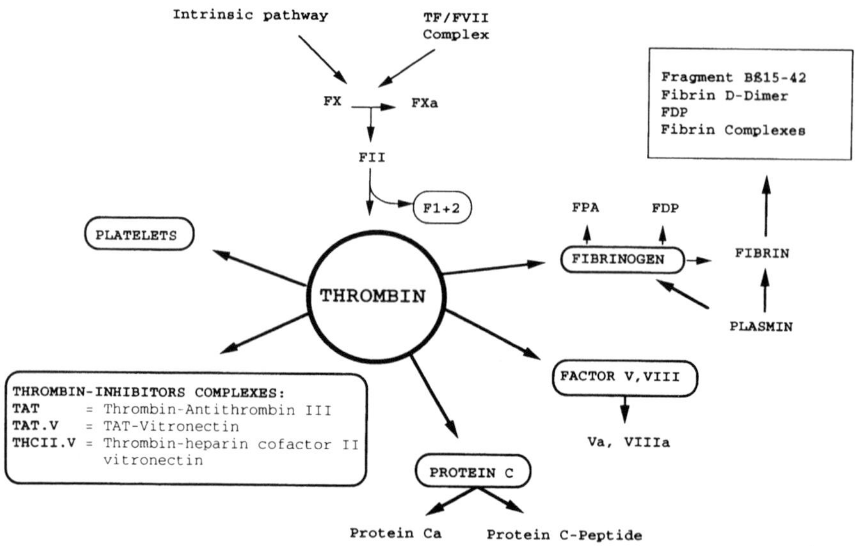

Figure 2. Schematic representation of the blood clotting system and inhibition mechanisms.

(THCII) complexes]. Further, plasmin produced in response to fibrin generation *in vivo* converts fibrinogen/fibrin into fibrinogen/fibrin degradation products (FDPs), including the D-dimer and the fibrin fragment b15-42. Elevation of the activation peptides, enzyme-inhibitors complexes and FDPs likely reflect increased *in vivo* coagulation.

Assays of plasma FPA, F1+2, TAT complex and D-dimer indicate that one or more of these parameters are increased in plasma of cancer patients. Thus, virtually all patients with leukemia or solid tumors, regardless of clinical evidence of TED, have laboratory signs indicative of increased clotting activation and fibrin production or low grade disseminated intravascular coagulation.[3,31]

In a recent study in 117 cancer patients undergoing surgery for localized tumors (mostly of the GI tract) we observed that the plasma levels of pre-operative TAT complex and F1+2 were significantly higher as compared to those in an age-matched control group of subjects ($p < 0.005$ and $p < 0.05$, respectively).[33] The pre-operative Factor VII concentrations were not significantly different (Table 1). Pre-surgical TAT levels ≥3.5 ng/ml also had a significant predictive value for post-operative deep vein thrombosis (DVT) in this group of patients. The calculated relative risk of having DVT in the single patient was 7.5 ($p < 0.01$, by Fisher's exact test).

Table 1
Pre-Surgical levels of plasma thrombin-antithrombin III (TAT), prothrombin fragment 1+2 (F1+2), zymogen factor VII (FVIIz) and total FVII (FVIIt) in cancer patients and healthy control subjects.

	CANCER PATIENTS (n=117)	CONTROLS (n=50)	p*
TAT (ng/ml)	2.7	2.3	<0.005
range	1.4 - 14.6	1.0 - 6.4	
F1+2 (nmol/l)	1,13	0,7	<0.05
range	0.4 - 16	0.34 - 1.45	
FVIIt (U/ml)	0.98	1.04	n.s.
range	0.59 - 1.45	0.73 - 1.42	
FVIIz (U/ml)	0.95	0.98	n.s.
range	0.4 - 1.54	0.57 - 1.74	

*Statistical comparisons made by the non-parametric Mann Whitney U test.

B. EVIDENCE FOR DECREASED THROMBIN INHIBITION

It has become important in this setting to establish whether the documented increase of thrombin production in malignancy is accompanied by a corresponding increase in thrombin inhibition, and whether the source of increased coagulation is intravascular, extravascular or both.

New studies are providing evidence which supports the concept that increased prothrombin activation in cancer is not paralleled by corresponding increases in the generation of thrombin-inhibitor complexes.[34] Prothrombinase converts prothrombin into equimolar concentration of thrombin and the stable peptide F1+2. The thrombin produced is readily inactivated by its major plasma inhibitors, ATIII and HCII, with the subsequent formation of the corresponding thrombin-inhibitor complexes.

To define the thrombin-inhibition potential and the major site of prothrombin activation *in vivo* in malignancy, we have measured the concentrations of F1+2 as an index of prothrombin activation *in vivo*, and the concentrations of binary TAT, ternary TAT.V and THCII.V complexes[35], as an index of thrombin inactivation in the plasmas of healthy volunteers (n = 37) and cancer patients (n = 39). The results of this preliminary study suggest that while the plasma levels of F1+2 of cancer patients are significantly greater than those of normal control subjects ($p < 0.001$), the levels of the thrombin-inhibitors complexes of these patients are decreased compared to the control group.[34] In normal plasma (where the concentrations of the four parameters likely reflect hemostasis), the sum of TAT, TAT.V and THCII.V was 61% of the levels of F1+2, compared with 30% in the plasmas of cancer patients (Fig. 3). Specifically, although binary TAT (which constitute less than 20% of TAT complexes in both groups) were found higher in cancer patients than in healthy subjects, the sum of the three parameters estimating thrombin inhibition in the cancer patients was only 30% that of F1+2, compared to 61% for normal individuals.

These observations raise the possibility that significant concentrations of thrombin escape inhibition in cancer. This free thrombin may represent an important aspect of the high risk for DVT associated with malignant disease.

IV. THERAPY

Prevention of thromboembolic complications in malignancy is warranted, given the evidence for a prothrombotic state. However, there are still no definite indications about the best prophylactic regimen(s) in these patients.

In surgical conditions, clinical trials evaluating different prophylactic methods have often included such a high risk group of cancer subjects although the study was not designed to assess the treatment in cancer patients.[3,23] In most instances low dose subcutaneous heparin or low molecular weight heparin have been safe and effective in reducing the rate of thrombosis in the patients whether or not they had cancer[3], consistent with a number of laboratory findings. In major surgery for cancer[34], as well as in other clinical conditions, such as major orthopedic surgery[36,37], there is an increase of binary TAT, which has been hypothesized to reflect an increase in intravascular coagulation associated with an increase in tissue factor availability. The plasma levels of TAT in the post-surgical cancer patients have been suppressed significantly by prophylactic doses of heparin or low molecular weight heparin, which also coincided with a reduced rate of DVT.[34,36,37]

In medical patients receiving outpatient chemotherapy, antithrombotic drugs (i.e. anticoagulants, in combination with fibrinolytics and antiplatelets) have been administered as adjunctive therapy for cancer in a number of different studies since 1976.[38] Warfarin has been proved to be effective to prolong significantly the survival of lung cancer patients in the VA CSP #75 study.[39] However, no conclusion can be drawn from this study concerning the prophylactic efficacy against thrombosis of any treatment regimens, since no objective criteria were defined to assess thrombosis clinically in the

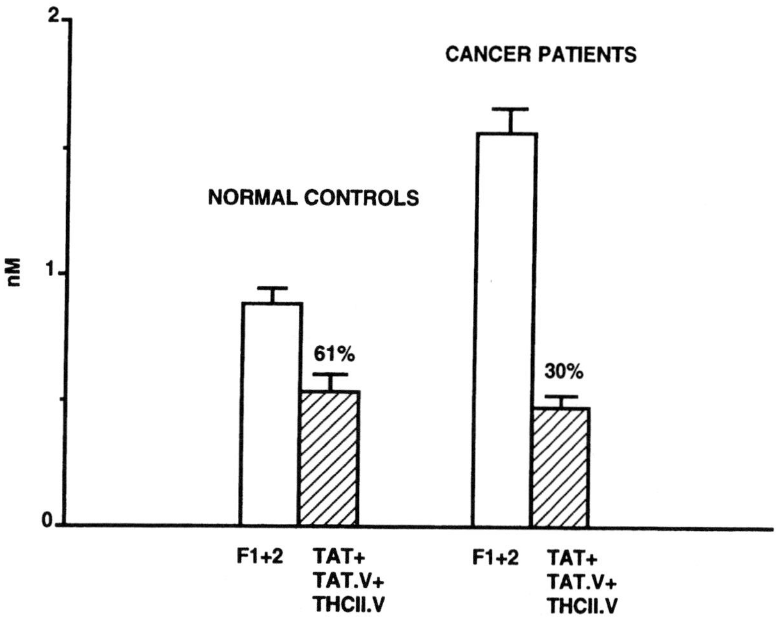

Figure 3. The sum of thrombin-inhibitor complexes expressed as a percentage of the total thrombin formed (estimated as F1+2). Comparison between healthy control subjects and cancer patients.

same group of individuals. The finding that FPA was significantly decreased ($p < 0.005$) in patients enrolled in the above cited VA CSP #75 study receiving warfarin is suggestive, however, that the prothrombotic potential was reduced in this patient group.[3,31] Recently, a randomized double blind trial of very low dose warfarin (PT INR range 1.3-1.9) in women receiving chemotherapy for stage IV breast cancer has been concluded. The results of this study demonstrate the safety and efficacy of this regimen, at least in this type of tumor.[40]

New approaches to preventing TED in cancer include the use of ATIII concentrates in some specific conditions, such as in acute lymphoblastic leukemia (ALL) patients during L-asparaginase therapy, a drug known to induce a hypercoagulable state.[26] Treatment with 50 U/Kg ATIII concentrates given to prevent DVT in these ALL patients, has been shown to reduce significantly the levels of markers of hypercoagulability, including F1+2 and binary TAT, with the simultaneous decrease of thromboembolic events.[41]

In conclusion, anticoagulant treatments remain a difficult task in cancer patients, particularly those who are also at high risk for bleeding. It may be more worthwhile to consider whether the main site of clotting activation in cancer patients actually occurs in the extravascular compartment. If so, it is possible that those drugs which are able to improve the natural anticoagulant property of the vessel wall, such as heparin and dermatan sulphate,[42] are potentially good candidates to prevent an early phase the prothrombotic process.

REFERENCES

1. **Donati, M.B., Poggi, A., Semeraro, N.** Coagulation and malignancy, In: *Recent Advances in Blood Coagulation*, Poller, L. (ed), Churchill Livingstone, London, 1981, pp 227.
2. **Rickles, F.R., Edwards, R.L.** Activation of blood coagulation in cancer: Trousseau's syndrome revisited. *Blood* 62, 14, 1983.
3. **Rickles, F.R., Levine, M.N., Edwards, R.L.** Hemostatic alterations in cancer patients. *Cancer Met Rev* 11, 237, 1992.
4. **Poggi, A., Donati, M.B., Garattini, S.** Fibrin and cancer cell growth: Problems in the evaluation of experimental models, In: *Malignancy and the Hemostatic System*, Donati, M.B., Davison, J.F., Garattini, S. (eds), Raven Press, New York, 1981, pp 89.
5. **Donati, M.B.** Hemostatic abnormalities in tumor-bearing animals, In: *Hemostatic Mechanisms and Metastasis*, Honn, K.V., Sloane, B.F. (eds), Martinus Nijhoff Publishing, Boston, 1984, pp 62.
6. **Bani, M.R., Falanga, A., Alessio, M.G., Radice, E., Consonni, R., Giavazzi, R., Donati, M.B.** Hemostatic changes in nude mice bearing human colon carcinomas (HCC) with different procoagulant capacity. *Int J Cancer* 50, 1, 1991.
7. **Ogura, T., Tsubura E., Yamamura, Y.** Localization of radioiodinated fibrinogen in invated and metastatized tumor tissue of Walker carcinosarcoma. *GANN* 61, 443, 1970.
8. **Robson, E.B., Murawski, G.F., Bettigole, R.E.** Use of 125I fibrinogen kinetic data to detect disseminated intravascular coagulation and deposition of fibrin in patients with metastatic cancer. *Thromb Haemost* 37, 484, 1977.
9. **Chew, E., Wallace, A.C.** Demonstration of fibrin in early stages of experimental metastases. *Cancer Res* 36, 1904, 1976.
10. **Peterson, H.I.** Fibrinolysis and antifibrinolytic drugs in the growth and spread of tumors. *Cancer Treat Rev* 4, 212, 1977.
11. **Ambrus, J.L., Ambrus, C.M., Gatspar, H.** Studies on platelet aggregation and platelet interaction with tumor cells, In: *Platelets: A Multidisciplinary Approach*, de Gaetano, G., Garattini, S. (eds), Raven Press; New York, 1978, pp 467.
12. **Gasic, G.J., Gasic, T.B., Galanti, N., Johnson, T., Murphy, S.** Platelet-tumor cell interactions in mice. The role of platelets in

the spread of malignant disease. *Int J Cancer* 11, 704, 1973.

13. **Colucci, M., Delaini, F., De Bellis Vitti, G., Locati, D., Poggi, A., Semeraro, N., Donati, M.B.** Warfarin inhibits both procoagulant activity and metastatic capacity of Lewis Lung Carcinoma cells: role of Vitamin K deficiency. *Biochem Pharmacol* 32, 1689, 1983.
14. **Pineo, J.F., Brian, M.C., Gallus, A.S., Hirsh, J., Hatton, M.W., Regoeczi, E.** Tumors mucus production, and hypercoagulability. *Ann NY Acad Sci* 230, 262, 1974.
15. **Bick, R.L.** Alterations of hemostasis associated with malignancy: Etiology, pathophysiology, diagnosis and management. *Semin Thromb Haemost* 5, 1, 1978.
16. **Sach, G.H., Jr., Levin, J., Bell, W.** Trousseau's syndrome and other manifestations of chronic disseminated coagulopathy in patients with neoplasms: Clinical, pathophysiologic and therapeutic features. *Medicine* 56, 1, 1977.
17. **Schafer, A.I.** Bleeding and thrombosis in the myeloproliferative disorders. *Blood* 64, 1, 1984.
18. **Cortelazzo, S., Viero, P., Finazzi, G., D'Emilio, A., Rodeghiero, F., Barbui, T.** Incidence and risk factors for thrombotic complications in an historical cohort of 100 patients with essential thrombocythemia. *J Clin Oncol* 8, 556, 1990.
19. **Falanga, A., Alessio, M.G., Donati, M.B., Barbui, T.** A new procoagulant in acute leukemia. *Blood* 71, 870, 1988.
20. **Alessio, M.G., Falanga, A., Consonni, R., Bassan, R., Minetti, B., Donati, M.B., Barbui, T.** Cancer procoagulant in acute lymphoblastic leukemia. *Eur J Haematol* 45, 78, 1990.
21. **Tallman, M.S., Kwaan, H.C.** Reassessing the hemostatic disorder associated with acute promyelocytic leukemia. *Blood* 79, 543, 1992.
22. **Rodeghiero, F., Avvisati, G., Castaman, G.C., Barbui T., Mandelli, F.** Early deaths and anti-hemorrhagic treatments in acute promyelocytic leukemia. *Blood* 75, 2112, 1990.
23. **Clagett, G.P., Reisch, J.S.** Prevention of venous thromboembolism in general surgical patients. *Ann Surg* 208, 227, 1988.
24. **Salzman, E.W., Hirsh, J.** Prevention of venous thromboembolism, In: *Hemostasis and Thrombosis. Basic Principles and Clinical Practice*, Colman, R.W., Marder, V.J., Salzman, E.W. (eds), J.B. Lippincott Company, Philadelphia, 1987, pp 1252.
25. **Levine, M.N., Gent, M., Hirsh, J., Arnold, A., Goodyear, M.D., DePauw, S.** The thrombogenic effect of anticancer drug therapy in women with stage II breast cancer. *N Engl J Med* 318, 404, 1988.
26. **Barbui, T., Finazzi, G., Donati, M.B., Falanga, A.** Antiblastic

therapy and thrombosis, In: *Thrombosis: An update*, Neri Serneri, G.G., Gensini, G.F., Abbate, R., Prisco, D. (eds), Scientific Press, Florence, 1992, pp 305.

27. **Prandoni, P., Lensing, A.W.A., Buller, H.R., Cogo, A., Prins, M.H., Cattelan, A.M., Cuppini, S., Noventa, F., ten Cate, J.W.** Deep vein thrombosis and the incidence of subsequent symptomatic cancer. *N Engl J Med* 327, 1128, 1992.
28. **Donati, M.B., Semeraro, N.** Cancer cell procoagulants and their pharmacological modulation. *Haemost* 14, 422, 1984.
29. **Nemerson, Y.** The tissue factor pathway of blood coagulation. *Semin Hematol* 29, 170, 1992.
30. **Falanga, A., Gordon, S.G.** Isolation and characterization of cancer procoagulant: A cysteine proteinase from malignant tissue. *Biochem* 24, 5558, 1985.
31. **Falanga, A., Barbui, T., Rickles, F.R., Levine, M.N.** Guidelines for clotting studies in cancer patients. *Thromb Haemost* 70, 540, 1993.
32. **Bauer, K.A., Rosenberg, R.D.** The pathophysiology of the prethrombotic state in humans: Insights gained from studies using markers of hemostatic system activation. *Blood* 70, 343, 1987.
33. **Falanga, A., Ofosu, F.A., Cortelazzo, S., Delaini, F., Consonni, R., Caccia, R., Longatti, S., Maran, D., Rodeghiero, F., Pogliani, E., Marassi, A., D'Angelo, A., Barbui, T.** Preliminary study to identify cancer patients at high risk for venous thrombosis following major surgery. *Br J Haematol* 85, 745, 1993.
34. **Falanga, A., Ofosu, F.A., Delaini, F., Oldani, E., Dewar, L., Lui, L., Barbui, T.** The hypercoagulable state in cancer patients: evidence for impaired thrombin inhibitions. *Blood Coag Fibrin*, 5 (Suppl 1), 519, 1994.
35. **Ofosu, F.A.** Personal communication.
36. **Ofosu, F.A., Leclerc, J., Delorme, F., Craven, S., Shafai, S., Frewin, L., Blajchman, M.A.** The low molecular weight heparin Enoxaparin inhibits the consumption of factor VII and prothrombin activation *in vivo* associated with elective knee replacement surgery. *Br J Haematol* 82, 391, 1992.
37. **Ofosu, F.A., Levine, M., Craven, S., Dewar, L., Shafai, S., Blajchman, M.A.** Prophylactically equivalent doses of Enoxaparin and unfractionated heparin inhibit *in vivo* coagulation to the same extent. *Br J Haematol* 82, 400, 1992.
38. **Zacharski, R.L., Donati, M.B.** Registry of clinical trials of antithrombotic drugs in cancer. *Thromb Haemost* 61, 526, 1989.
39. **Zacharski, R.L., Henderson, W.G., Rickles, F.R., Forman, W.B.,**

Cornell, C.J., Forcier, R.J., Edwards, R.L., Headley, E., Kim, S.H., O'Donnell, J.F., O'Dell, R., Tornyos, K., Kwaan, H.C. Effect of Warfarin anticoagulation on survival in carcinoma of the lung, colon, head and neck and prostate: Final report of VA Cooperative Study #75. *Cancer* 53, 2046, 1984.

40. **Levine, M.N., Hirsh, J., Gent, M., Arnold, A., Warr, D., Falanga, A., Samosh, M., Bramwell, W., Pritchard, K., Stewart, D., Goodwin, P., Dickson, L.** A double blind randomized trial of mini-dose warfarin for the prevention of thromboembolism in patients with stage IV breat cancer. *Thromb Haemost* 69, 981, 1993.

41. **Mazzucconi, M.G., Cugliotta, L., Leone, G., Dragoni, F., Mattioli Belmonte, M., DeStefano, V., Chistolini, A., Tura, S., Mandelli, F.** Antithrombin III infusion suppresses the hypercoagulable state in adult acute lymphoblastic leukemia patients treated with low dose of E. coli L-asparaginase: a GIMENA study. *Blood Coag Fibrinolysis*, In press, 1994.

42. **Cortellazo, S., Buchanan, M.R., Young, E., Hirsh, J., Van Ryn-McKenna, J., Ofosu, F.A.** Continous infusion of low affinity heparin and dermatan sulphate induce the release into rabbit blood of a moiety which catalyzes thrombin-antithrombin III formation. *Thromb Haemorrh Dis* 2/1, 17, 1990.

INDEX